<u>Diabetic Diary</u>

<u>An Ordinary Type 2 Diabetic Patient's</u>

<u>Ridiculous Charting Challenge</u>

<u>to Control Blood Sugar and</u>

<u>Stop Insulin in 30 Days</u>

by Cheryl Pouhl

Dedicated to my current and former physicians

who have tried their best

for a bad patient.

Disclaimer

This book is a personal journal of an ordinary patient. I am not a physician. I do not make any warranty, express or implied or assume any legal responsibility for the accuracy, completeness, or usefulness of my methods. The information in the book should not be a substitute for your personal physician's professional advice. The author disclaims any responsibility for problems that may occur by following the information in this text.

Diabetic Diary

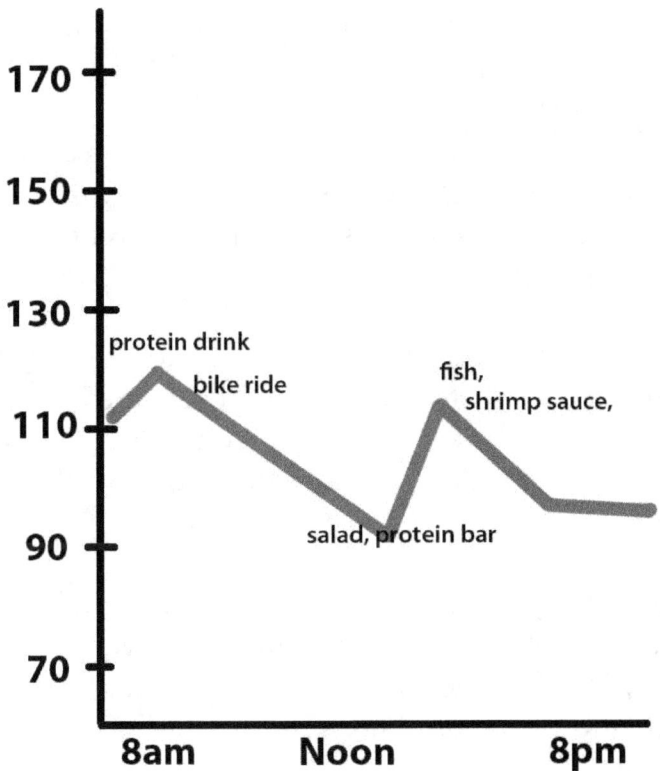

Foreword

I hope the detailed personal information in this book is useful to readers. I kept a record of 30 days of diet, exercise and medication changes in my battle to overcome type 2 diabetes. I encountered many surprises during the frequent blood sugar charting challenge. Most of the surprises were the result of mistakes in the recommendations given by diabetic authorities.

I detail the conversation with my doctor that finally inspired me to take responsibility. I chart the day to day food choices and the objective outcome. In spite of my stubborn will and refusal to respond to failure I had some success.

Within 30 days I had ceased needing or using insulin. Within 60 days I had lost 16 pounds. However, within 120 days my blood sugar was creeping upward again along with a few pounds. This is a war without an end.

Is this a how-to book? *Definitely not.* This is how I won a battle in spite of my errors. I hope the reader will learn from my mistakes.

Chapter One

The Promise and the Problem of a Bad Patient

... I could not control my hunger and overeating until I knew my sugar levels and could differentiate high glucose craving from low glucose hunger...

I have always been skeptical and needed personal proof through testing and often failure. I am an exceedingly bad patient and resistant to lifestyle change. Perhaps this is because my other medical issues have seemed to eventually disappear with time and no treatment. *Ignore it and it will go away, I believed.*

I found education on diabetes was both plentiful and deficient. Outdated and disproven recommendations were repeatedly suggested in diabetic menus. The diabetic authorities and major medical centers are resistant to changing their traditional diabetic diets based on old concepts and overly concerned with general health.

A well respected medical center diabetic recommendations included; whole wheat pancakes, carrots, cottage cheese, beans, peas and fruit. These are all food items that my self testing revealed I could not eat without dramatic increase in my blood sugar.

Diabetic education classes were too elementary and unprepared fellow participants delayed progress toward mastering the information. Physicians have the detailed scientific information but not the time required, so education is outsourced.

The result is an entire type 2 diabetic patient population inundated with ineffective and irrelevant recommendations on websites that claim credibility. Insulin and blood sugar recommendations are largely directed at those with type 1 diabetes, not type 2. Most adult patients are type 2, usually caused by lifestyle habits.

I know the common wisdom and evidence is that weight gain leads to type 2 diabetes. *I wonder, instead, if the increasing glucose levels during pre-diabetes leads to overeating and weight gain.*

I could not control my hunger and overeating until I knew my sugar levels and could differentiate high glucose craving from low glucose hunger. The symptoms felt the same to me. Only with my Charting Challenge frequent sugar monitoring could I see the proof of whether I was **craving food or actually hungry**. I could respond appropriately when I knew my glucose level.

July 27 2015- The Motivating Scolding and Promise

It started with a promise to my new doctor. It began with a detailed interview of what I ate for breakfast and lunch. I recall thinking to myself, *("Don't you have other patients waiting? Is this really important?")* Ultimately it was a most useful time spent because I realized if it was important enough for him, it needed to be important to me.

I told him all of the items I thought I ate. His honest and hurtful response, "If you really ate like this why aren't you skinny?"

"Exactly" I replied while self examining my choices and my weight. I realized I knew what to eat but when I recorded everything that went into my mouth it was alarming.

He raised further questions about my exercise schedule. He was genuinely shocked that I rode my bike 15 miles. "How often do you do that?"

"Four times a week" and often more than that, I thought.

"But only when it is warm out." He persisted still not acknowledging I could be in good condition. I was obviously overweight. "If you didn't bike you would be seriously ill", he scolded.

"What is your blood sugar two hours after you eat?" he demanded.

I searched my memory when I had last measured it two hours after I ate. It was weeks, perhaps months earlier.

"170?" I guessed meekly, wondering if it was a good number.

"170?" He asked with contempt. He didn't seem very impressed.

"Promise me you will eat better." He repeated the demand three times.

"I promise. I promise. I promise." I used to be in professional sales. He used a perfect close. I knew I would keep my word. If any physician reads this book, I would advise they respond to patients in this way.

"140 blood sugar two hours after you eat, 100-110 in the morning. If it spikes too low or high call me." He sent me off.

I am sure I have been told before what the numbers should be, I just never remembered. This was a conversation I would never forget.

Eight Years of Living With Type 2 Diabetes

I always felt God punishes me for insensitive thoughts about others and I have numerous examples. For years, while I was skinny I dismissed type 2 diabetes as not a real disease. I wondered why overweight people just didn't quit eating until they were skinny. *Yes, I am cruel!*

I was diagnosed eight years earlier with type 2 diabetes at age 54. My A1C at the time was over 11 and I was seriously hyperglycemic. Until July 2015, I had A1C's measure between 5.9 to 6.8. At one time, 7.8, after an entire season of a poorly treated bladder infection

My previous doctor had seemed moderately satisfied with my A1C numbers until recently. At the last appointment she told me to increase the insulin to bring fasting levels down to 110. She suggested increasing doses by 2 units until fasting levels returned to 110.

My A1C history from the time I was first diagnosed with type 2 diabetes is on the following chart. During the first six months I made great progress. My progress stalled until I started the challenge recorded in this text. A1C's of 4-6 are considered great by some diabetic authorities. Normal is about 5.5.

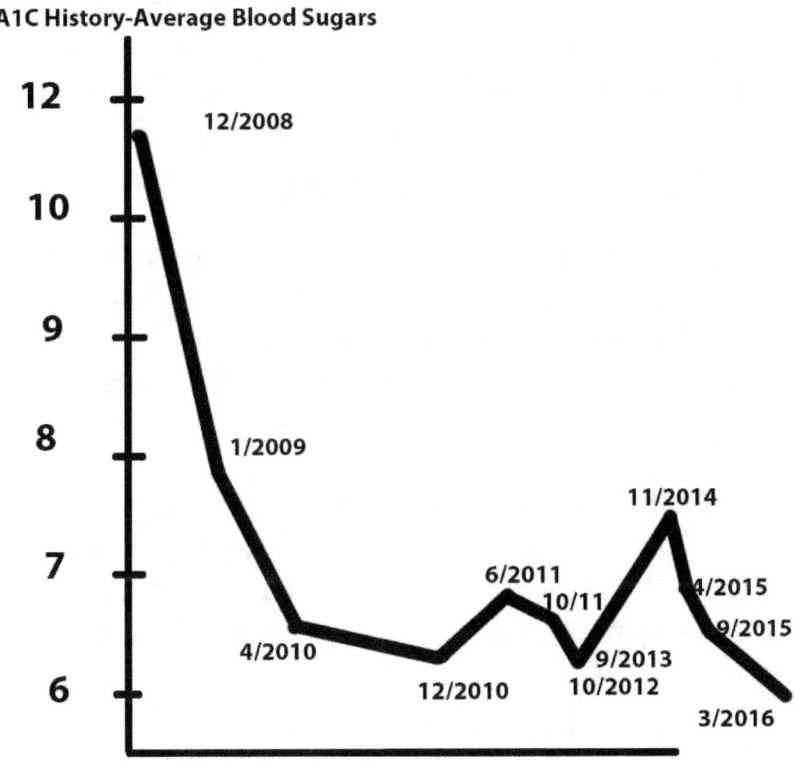

A1C History-Average Blood Sugars

She didn't realize I wasn't motivated enough. When I attempted to control diabetes through long term insulin I sometimes reached 24 units and my sugar was still resistant to treatment. She eventually prescribed a short term insulin also. I never understood how to combine the two insulin types with success. I always feared low sugars.

Suspect Authority. I found one well recognized medical authority offer diabetic recommendations as 90-130 sugars before meals and 180 sugars 1-2 hours after meals. These levels are too high for type 2 diabetics! The same authority included fat free ice cream and cocoa mix in their food recommendations for diabetic patients. *Yikes!*

Blood sugar goals stated for non diabetics at a recognized diabetic education I found more appropriate for my type 2 diabetics. Less than 110 before lunch, supper or snack, less than 100 before breakfast, less than 140 two hours after a meal and less than 120 at bedtime.

I usually settled on about 14 units a day of long term insulin during the past eight years because I knew it was insufficient to cause low sugar in the afternoons. By dosing low I didn't have to worry about monitoring for hypoglycemia.

I rarely measured my blood sugar. My test strips went bad from advanced age in my closet. My fasting glucose in the morning was typically 120-130. I didn't worry, I knew about the *dawn effect* and my glucose was lower in the afternoon.

Dawn Effect; in some diabetic patients blood sugar increases between 2 and 8 AM. It may be due to hormone production overnight affecting insulin levels, or a carbohydrate snack late at night.

I could often tell it took a long time for the blood sugar high symptoms to diminish after larger meals. Many diabetic patients have delayed stomach emptying. It is common in diabetics and may be due to high glucose damage to nerves in the stomach.

I sometimes woke in the night with a racing heart and high sugar from a late snack. Some medical authorities believe sleep disruption interferes with the bodies repair mechanism and leads to obesity and diabetes. *I wonder if instead, high blood sugar leads to chronic sleep disruption.*

Family Inheritance

Diabetes is apparently my inheritance. Both of my brothers were diagnosed with diabetes the same year as me. My grandfather was on insulin for decades. My father, a chronic smoker all of his life, escaped the disease. My brother was hospitalized after an emergency visit. His wife was told he probably had TB or lung cancer. Actually his lungs were filled with fungus. As I sat with my very ill brother in the ICU, I noticed a nurse giving him insulin. His blood sugar was over 1000! I advised the nurse that my brother never was diagnosed with diabetes.

They discharged him a week later from the hospital with a brown bag full of insulin and needles. This was a man who could never even force himself to insert a contact lens! He never did learn to use insulin but he is now stable on oral medication and daily exercise.

My younger brother never saw a doctor either so I tested his blood sugar in our hotel room on a visit to his hometown. His glucose was over 500! Just like me, he had no idea or symptoms. He also had no insurance or doctor. He was initially treated with insulin by his daughter's kind and compassionate clinic pediatrician.

My brother then read the <u>Dr Bernstein's Diabetes Solution: A Complete Guide to Achieving Normal Blood Sugars</u> [1] book that I sent him. This book is useful because Dr. Bernstein wrote about his personal experience as a type 1 diabetes patient. My brother was able to stop insulin treatment based on a careful diet of controlling carbohydrates. *He was always smarter than me.*

Bad Habits

I was a ballet and toe dancer for twenty years and kept a skinny figure no matter what I ate. I weighed 105 to 115 pounds for 35 years. I had to intentionally overeat so that I could donate blood. When I was a student I bought a decorated birthday cake to eat every week. After a few weeks the bakery staff quit asking if I wanted to add a name to the cake decoration. *Just hand over the pretty cake to the skinny girl!* Occasionally I added potato chips and onion dip with a coke to my diet.

---

[1] Bernstein, Richard K MD, <u>Dr Bernstein's Diabetes Solution: A Complete Guide to Achieving Normal Blood Sugars</u>, Little, Brown and Co., 1997

I admit I have an emotional attachment to birthday cakes, especially with brightly colored roses.

For the next twenty eight years I gained 1 1/2 pounds a year. It was too little for me to notice. Clothes that no longer fit were ready to be replaced. I noticed visible fat for the first time in a clothes store fitting room. My perfect husband never spoke negatively about my weight gain while his weight remained the same since college. I would tease him, "Do you want a skinny wife or a happy wife?." *He always made the wise choice.*

When we married, he convinced me to eat breakfast for the first time in my life and regular meals for my health. We ate an unsweetened breakfast cereal and toast in the morning. For lunch we would have a small turkey and cheese sandwich. We would often follow meals with yogurt. These were considered healthy meal options. We had no idea the cereal, toast, sandwiches and even the yogurt would have negative consequences for me.

Weight Loss as A Motivator

I have read that type 2 diabetics are insulin resistant, not insulin deficient. Added weight increases the resistance but weight loss reduces resistance and increases insulin sensitivity.

Glucose levels increase in the blood in type 2 diabetes when there is insulin resistance. Exercise makes cells more sensitive to insulin. Fat cells are more resistant to insulin.

Since a side effect of high insulin levels is increased weight around the abdomen I was anxious to reduce insulin. As an added benefit it was far easier to lose weight after I maintained steady blood sugars and stopped the insulin.

 The focus of my journal was not about my weight; however, 16 pounds were lost in 60 days by monitoring and controlling my blood sugar. By day 25 I had already lost 9 pounds. Recently I read a diabetic authority telling patients to keep the carbohydrate intake in their diet constant so that the insulin remains constant. *I am sure glad I was never given that advice.*

Even Non Diabetics Should Have a Blood Sugar Test Kit.

I read that eight years before diagnosis those with type 2 diabetes already have lost a significant number of pancreatic cells from high glucose toxicity.

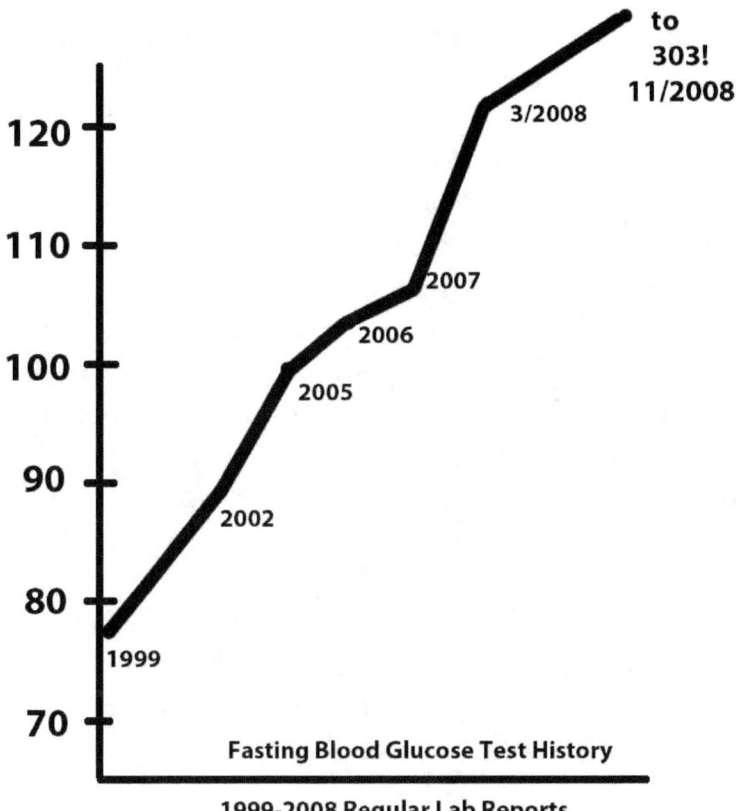

My Fasting Glucose Levels on Lab Tests from 1999 to Diagnosis of Diabetes in 2008

to 303! 11/2008

3/2008

120

110

2007

100

2006

2005

90

2002

80

1999

70

Fasting Blood Glucose Test History

1999-2008 Regular Lab Reports

How was my rising blood glucose missed? My lab records reveal increasing fasting blood sugars for nine years before my diagnosis when it reached 303! I didn't recognize any symptoms at the time.

I now encourage all of my friends to buy a blood sugar test kit from the pharmacy and occasionally test their sugar. Do not rely on recognizing the gradual symptoms. Years ago I read that pregnant women who have gestational diabetes will likely be diagnosed with diabetes a decade later. Gestational diabetes (diabetes during pregnancy) often results in babies weighing over 10 pounds.

The blood sugar test kits cost only $20 and it only takes a minute. I agree the instructions for the kits should be simpler. My husband, an engineer, and myself, a former health consultant, wasted many test strips while learning the testing method. Some require a drop of blood be placed on the side instead of the end of the strip. The timing is critical, you must be prepared, poked and ready with a drop of blood, before you insert the test strip into the tester. The blood drop should be upright before touching it with the testing portion of the paper strip. Remove your finger as soon as the dashes appear in the test window. If you have too little or too much blood on the strip it will ruin the test.

I discovered that by ordering test strips on amazon.com the cost was far less than at retail. Only 16 cents per strip allowed me to test repeatedly with less concern for the cost. I used to spend $1 per strip.

My First Time

In the first ten days after my diagnosis my fasting glucose dropped from 396 to 146 through omission of sweets and taking the oral anti glycemic drug. The effect of the medication and diet change began to take effect after three days. I have continued to find a three day window before major changes appear in my glucose level.

I had symptoms of fatigue during this time due to the sudden reduction in what had become my normal glucose level. I was off to a great start but the reductions never went any father.

I had to switch from the oral anti-glycemic to insulin due to liver enzyme elevations. At the time my fasting sugar was 146. A month after using 10 units of long term insulin my fasting sugars were still 110 to 140. It didn't change significantly over the following eight years.

My first insulin injection occurred in a hotel room on the drive to Florida. The thought of injecting into my stomach still causes me revulsion. I have never permitted my husband to observe.

Fortunately, I had a dog with diabetes years earlier and had learned to inject him with insulin twice a day in the back of the neck. I used the same technique by squeezing a handful of skin and underlying fat and injecting at an angle.

I have always been very careful with disposing of needles. When I supervised a public health department we routinely dealt with garbage collectors who were accidentally punctured by loose needles.

I was told to use the insulin at night but I worried about sugars getting too low while I slept. I injected it in the morning so that I could observe the effects while awake.

On occasion, after reading diabetic management books I would achieve good sugar control through diet. My self control was usually erased in only a few days after social engagements, family celebrations and restaurant meals.

I often noticed that some vials or packages of insulin didn't seem to be as effective as others. Frequently the effectiveness of the first vial in the shipment was noticeably better than the last vial in the shipment. My mail order pharmacy sometimes sent the insulin in an insulated envelope with freezer packs. Once it was on my door step in subzero temperatures and another time in summer heat.

Diabetic Diets and Confusion

I had not acknowledged the connection between carbohydrates and blood sugar until after this 30 day challenge. I discovered the connection months later and realized my blood sugar testing had resulted in a personal low carb diet. It made me curious about recommendations I had apparently missed. However, the CDC site recommends a diabetic diet with less meat and more whole grain cereals, rice, bread and bagels. Bagels contain 60 grams of carbs! Oatmeal has 27 grams in a half cup serving! White rice has about 50 carbohydrates per cup, brown rice has 35 grams in a half cup. Whole grain flour has 86 grams of flour, compared to 95 grams of white flour per cup! *None of these seem like reasonable choices for diabetics.*

One diabetic authority reported that **vegetables contribute little carbohydrate and are not counted**. I have had to completely eliminate many vegetables from my diet, based on my glucose testing. A single carrot can contain 5 grams of carbs. Brussel sprouts have 11 grams and peas, 10 grams of carbohydrates. I sometimes include these in meals but I realize I have to balance a reduction elsewhere. My primary side vegetable in recent weeks is green beans at 5 grams per 1/2 cup.

Some diabetic authorities recommend vegetables like carrots, sweet potatoes, and many beans. **I followed their advice on sweet potatoes for eight years. Recently I found that a sweet potato, at 22 grams actually has higher carbohydrates than a small white potato at 15 grams.**

I understand that they are recommending a well rounded diet for the benefit of other health consequences of diabetes. The problem of their well meaning intentions is that the blood sugar in susceptible diabetics is more likely to be uncontrolled. I reason that I can address diet insufficiencies with vitamins, minerals and oil supplements while still focusing on my sugar. *What do I know? I am only a patient.*

They caution diabetic patients against changing their meal time or quantity because it would affect the insulin dose! *Shouldn't improvement be the goal?*

A diabetic authority referenced an example of a diabetic patient needing 75 grams of carbohydrates for breakfast each day! *How large is this patient?* The same authority cautioned against the danger of too much protein or fat in the diet...*but 75 grams of carbs is okay for breakfast?*

I found one diabetes education site that admitted that no one meal plan is for everyone. *Maybe they realize they are wrong? Perhaps I am carbohydrate intolerant?*

The diabetic authority admitted that cholesterol, sodium, fats, and calories were considered in their diet selections. *I thought so!*

They also admit that total carbohydrate counting is the first tool as a stronger predictor of blood glucose than glycemic index. *I knew it!*

In the same search I found a major medical center website that said the amount of carbohydrate is less important than the type of carbohydrate. *Not according to my tests!*

…Only with my Charting Challenge frequent sugar monitoring could I see the proof of whether I was craving food or actually hungry. I could respond appropriately when I knew my glucose level…

Chapter Two

The Necessity of my Charting Challenge

...What I learned immediately was that I couldn't tell anything based on how I felt...

Blood Sugar Testing To Determine Food Choices and Timing

I realized that only I had the ability to constantly test my blood sugar. Decisions on insulin and diet could only be made by myself on a daily basis. Diabetic authorities had lost credibility with me.   I used the self test meter and kept a vial of test strips and meters with me in my purse, car and at home. I tested every morning, and intended to test after lunch, dinner and before bedtime. *Eventually it hardly hurts at all.*

 What I learned immediately was that I couldn't tell anything based on how I felt. **The symptoms of low blood sugar and high blood sugar felt the same to**

me. On occasion I felt fine but the test revealed my sugar was high. Food cravings usually indicated my blood sugar was high, but occasionally also low. It was impossible to manage my diabetes without the tester. After observing the blood sugar results for days and seeing some patterns I introduced my own strategy.

If I didn't eat until my blood sugar was less than 110, my blood sugar was better controlled. I only followed this rule on the days at the end of the challenge because of my original concern of low sugar levels. For the same reason, while still taking insulin, I did not use it unless my blood glucose was at least 110.

Based on the testing I learned that larger meals, even those relatively small compared to the past, raised my blood sugar too much. It didn't matter that they were composed of low glycemic foods. If there was too much food of any type, my blood sugar went too high. A half order of chicken breast salad was usually okay. A full order of salad was too much.

July 28 2015, The Beginning

I imagined my recent renewed campaign against diabetes as a D-Day launch of war. My father fought as a paratrooper at D-Day. I could win my pathetic lifestyle war against type 2 diabetes.

It was a horrible time to start a new diabetic diet. In a few days I would go to Florida and prepare a vacation for our grandchildren who would arrive within a week. However, the time alone without food in the seasonal house would be welcome. Perhaps this experience would be instructive to the reader. Begin the challenge wherever you are. There will never be the perfect setting.

Frequent glucose testing and constant monitoring of my food intake was required for me to understand how little food created so much sugar.

I had eaten in the past to match my husband's eating pattern even if I didn't feel like eating. Now I could justify that my blood sugars were too high to eat another meal again. It took the burden from me of eating when I wasn't hungry.

... I wonder based on my personal experience if the increasing glucose levels during pre-diabetes leads to overeating and weight gain...

This approach for diabetics will not work for non-diabetics, whose blood sugar remains steady. It is one useful aspect of diabetes, an objective diet control tool.

Just like my experience when first diagnosed with diabetes, there was about a three day delay in response to my diet and medication changes. The glucose response to changes in my diet became less resistant to change as my challenge proceeded. I hope this insight is useful to the reader.

I have read that chronic exposure to elevated glucose and free fatty acids causes pancreatic beta cell damage. In type 2 diabetes some beta cells are active and repairable if high glucose damage is controlled.

Indigestion, Acid Reflux and Inappropriate Treatment

During this time of dietary changes I had frequent bouts of indigestion. My doctor explained that the pancreas has two major functions, exocrine and endocrine, one affecting digestive enzymes and the other hormones like insulin. It seemed reasonable to me that if my pancreas was impaired I would have symptoms of both.

I used several over the counter remedies to address the symptoms. My doctor advised me not to allow repeated attacks of acid reflux because of the potential esophageal cancer risk. Since that time I prevent acid reflux with acid reducers and inhibitors when they occur and now, months later, rarely have acid attacks.

Diet Experimentation Based on Blood Sugar Testing

I didn't realize until months later that I was practicing a low carb diet. I learned through the self testing challenge that a piece of meat, or vegetable, without being mixed with a carbohydrate filler like potatoes, sauce, soup, bread or rice was the best glucose limiting diet. It is not possible for me to eat too much food unless it is mixed with carbohydrates like potatoes, bread or rice. Without the added starches, I would gladly refrigerate half the meat portion for another meal.

I was surprised to discover that large salads affected my blood sugar. Later I learned that fresh vegetables in large portions have too many carbohydrates. My salads continue to be side salad portions. Even the balsamic vinaigrette dressings, as many others, are loaded with carbohydrates. A restaurant that promotes their salads recently placed their popular salad dressing in retail stores. A primary ingredient was high fructose corn syrup, which has a most powerful impact on my blood sugar. Surprisingly, blue cheese is my best option as a salad dressing to restrict carbohydrates.

A recognized diabetic authority recommended 45-60 carbs **per meal**. I found success reducing glucose only by limiting foods that contain about 50 grams carbs **per day.**

Before Charting

I had kept notes with dates and sugar levels on occasion for years. They were written in log books and kept in my bathroom drawer, desk, car, kitchen, never to be read or analyzed again. They were old news. *I was always expecting to be thinner and healthier tomorrow.*

The Charting

My notes were useful for the day but I realized I needed some organization to review longer term trends. I used to be a sales consultant and we relied on visual aids for quick and effective presentations.

I created my Charting Challenge to organize all the loose papers with critical information.

I created a template and recorded daily readings across the graph depicting the range of my blood sugars throughout the day. I always measured it on waking and usually two hours after I ate and bedtime. On some occasions I would measure the afternoon lows. I charted every day for two months. My original graphs are by hand. The first 30 days are presented in the next chapter. After this time the charts revealed a more steady blood sugar pattern. *I have included a template for the reader to copy and use on the last page.*

The Charting had another benefit, I could visualize my future chart and how the potential food selection would affect my graph.   Sometimes it was a valuable tool to avoid cheating. As I have noted, negative eating could affect my sugars for a few days.

Meal Timing Based on My Charting

If I ate too soon after the previous meal I would have a rapid and long lasting spike in blood sugar.   I believe that my system requires far longer than others to digest food, because of delayed stomach emptying. Sometimes I wake up still full from a dinner 12 hours earlier.

The charting allowed me objective measures for food selection and meal timing.

Glycemic Index and Net Carbs Was Ineffective Compared to Total Carbohydrates

Months after my challenge I realized carbs were the answer. I had read about the GI -Glycemic Index scale. Glycemic index tables calculated and ranked foods relative to the effect of white bread. It seemed so scientific and proven but also confusing. Low glycemic foods had scores below 55. They included whole wheat, pumpernickel bread, oatmeal, pasta of rice or barley, sweet potatoes, corn, butter beans, and most fruits.

High glycemic foods are rated with scores of 70 and above. They are white bread, cornflakes, white rice macaroni and cheese, potato, popcorn, pretzel, and pumpkin.

I would find that the total carbohydrate counts were the best indicator of effect on my blood sugar based on my self testing.

The same failed result occurred with net carbs, a newer standard by adjusting carbs based on fiber content. In my experience products with low net carbs produced the same glucose as the total carbohydrate indicated it would. For months I rode my bike for 15 miles and ate an energy bar with low net carbs. The bike rides had little effect on my weight or reduction of sugar until I quit eating an energy bar.

Insulin Increase Experiment

Based on the recommendation of my prior doctor, I experimented with increasing my insulin to lower my sugar. I increased my morning and evening injections of long acting insulin from the first day. It failed to produce the dramatic results I expected.

Insulin Reduction

Too low of blood sugar for insulin treatment was rarely an issue in the previous eight years. After about ten days monitoring sugar and adjusting my diet I sometimes avoided insulin because I worried that my sugar would get too low. I decided I would not use insulin if my sugar measured 110 or less. Within thirty days I had ceased using insulin entirely. Because of my ignorance I never considered simply reducing the insulin dose slowly.

The reader would probably be advised by their physician to adjust the insulin downward slowly.

I had discovered a year before my Charting Challenge that a prolonged bladder infection had raised my sugar to over 300 on some days. I do not know if it was due to the pain, stress or the infection. Since that time when I have an unusually high sugar level I consider if I might have an infection. Overall health is important to controlling sugar and sugar control is important to overall health. Infections are more likely when sugar is high because the immune system is more susceptible.

Chapter Three

The 30 Day Diary

and Charting

... I was consistently surprised how long it takes to reduce sugar levels and how little food it takes to raise sugar levels. ...

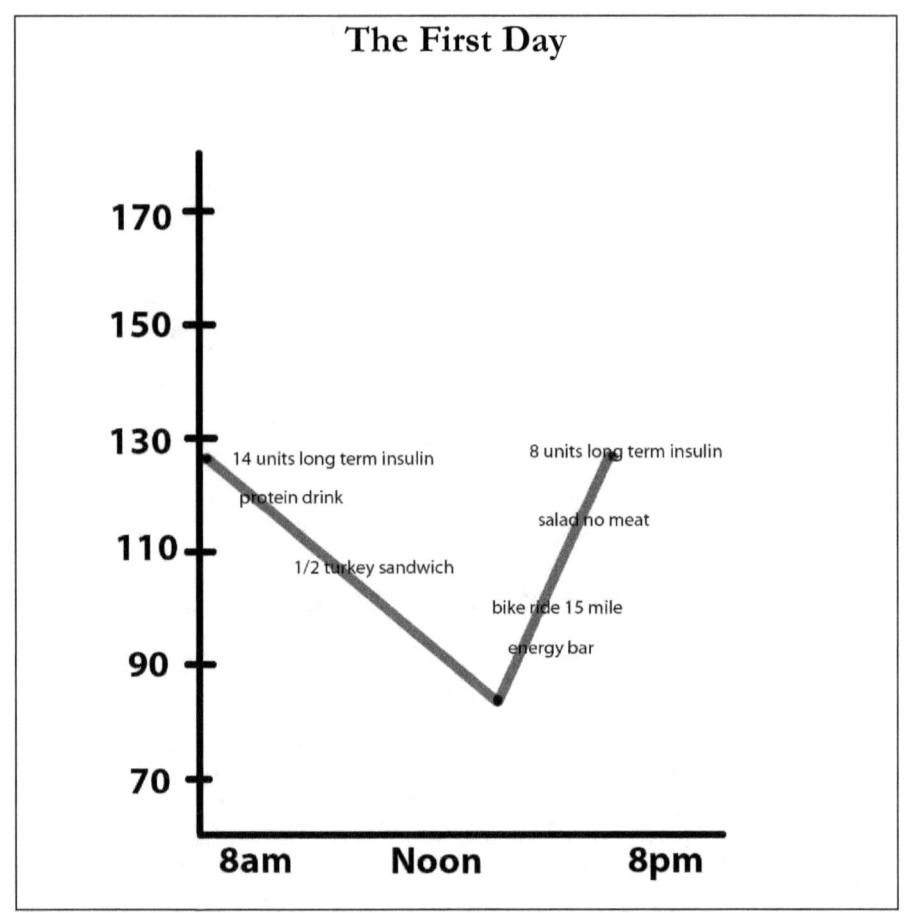

The First Day

170	
150	
130	14 units long term insulin
	protein drink
110	1/2 turkey sandwich
90	
70	

8 units long term insulin

salad no meat

bike ride 15 mile

energy bar

8am   Noon   8pm

The first day my fasting blood sugar was high and typical, at 127. I decided to follow my prior physician's advice and increase my insulin to keep my fasting sugar below 110. I injected more insulin than normal today. I also restricted my diet substantially this day but the sugar still rebounded. Later I would realize that the sugar stays in my system for about three days. I was surprised that the long bike ride had no impact on my sugar. I didn't realize until months later that the protein energy bars I often ate on the rides contained too many carbohydrates.

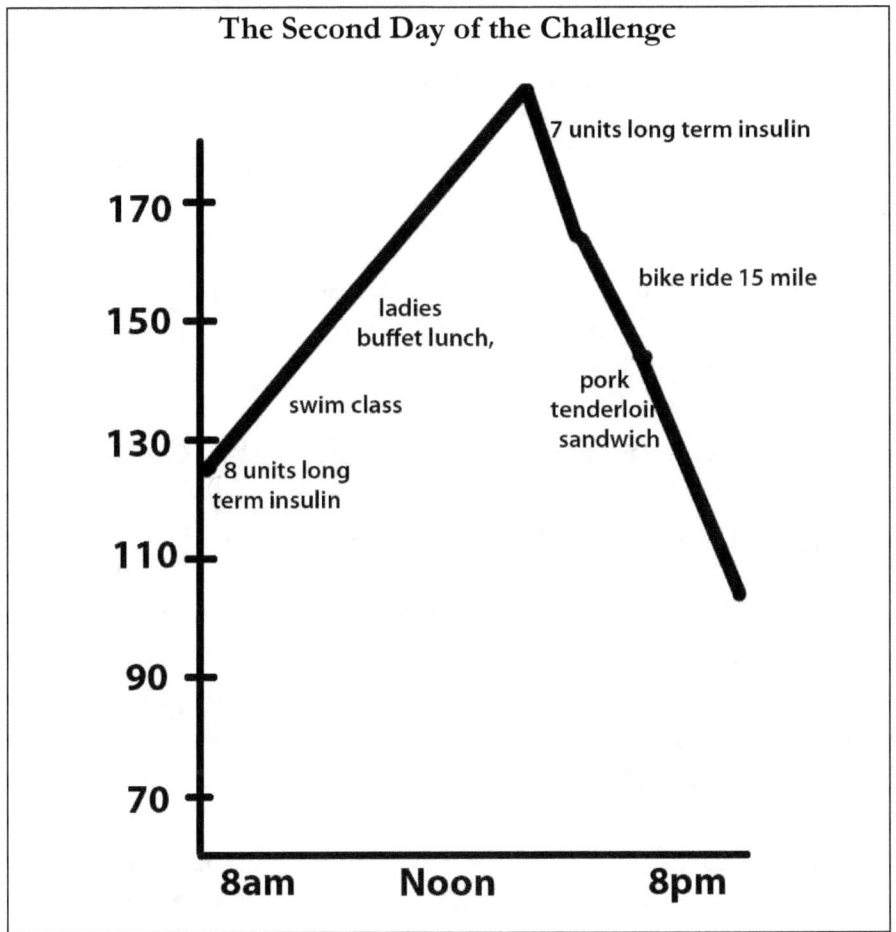

The Second Day of the Challenge

I was expecting my fasting blood sugar to be low this morning after the insulin injection last night. Instead it was the same, 127. "Was the insulin not working?" I remember reading once that the optimal maximum dose of insulin was 7 units. Still depending on the insulin, I divided my future doses. I injected 8 units of long acting insulin before I attended a ladies luncheon buffet. I selected mostly from the salad section and added a few tortilla chips and salsa. Two hours later my sugar was very high at 190. I was still unaware at the time of the high carbohydrate content of salad ingredients.

Salad dressings sometimes had sugar or high fructose corn syrup as a top ingredient, even a vinaigrette style dressing. I no longer expect low blood glucose results after salad choices.

I took 7 more units of long acting insulin and at 4 PM I was surprised it was still 160. I didn't realize how long it takes to purge my system of sugars.

We took our standard 15 mile bike ride and to our usual destination, a small rural bar. I thought my blood sugar must be low after extra insulin and the bike ride.

On the bike ride, we ordered a pork tenderloin sandwich with no fries, the healthiest item on the menu. At 7 PM, I was surprised my sugar was 137. An hour later, finally the blood sugar dropped to 105. Was this a delayed reaction to the extra insulin?

I was surprised that the long bike rides did not have more of an impact on my blood sugar. **Later I would read that weight lifting burns 19 times more insulin than aerobic activity.** The frequency of our bike riding and the uniformity of our regular route also probably factored in the minimal impact. **The efficacy of weight lifting in sugar reduction was confirmed in my self testing.**

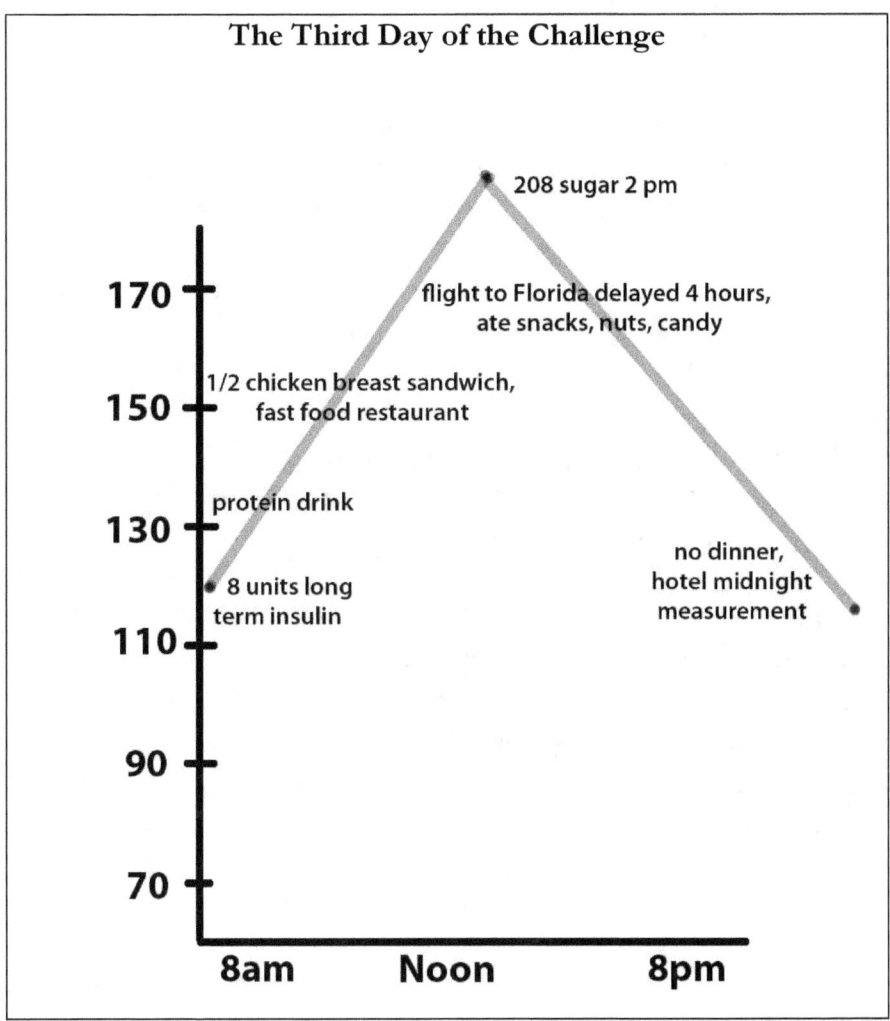

The Third Day of the Challenge

208 sugar 2 pm

flight to Florida delayed 4 hours,
ate snacks, nuts, candy

1/2 chicken breast sandwich,
fast food restaurant

protein drink

8 units long
term insulin

no dinner,
hotel midnight
measurement

170

150

130

110

90

70

8am   Noon   8pm

The following morning my blood sugar was 123. It had risen almost 20 points overnight! I read that the liver produces glucose during the night as a result of pancreatic hormones. It is called the *dawn effect.* I took 8 units of long acting insulin and a protein powder and meal replacement that boasted a healthy and low glycemic response.

For lunch my husband and I shared a broiled chicken sandwich at a popular fast food restaurant. At 2 PM my sugar was 208! The sandwich was the healthiest and newest item on the menu. I wondered how high other menu sandwiches would have caused my sugar level. I thought about another family member with type 2 diabetes that regularly eats at that fast food restaurant.

Today is the day that I fly to Florida alone, perhaps I am stressed? Later I would realize that high stress usually increases my sugar by about 50 points.

My early evening flight was four hours late. Only a snack bar was open in the regional airport. I bought a bag of peanuts and peanut M&M's.

I arrived in Florida at 1 AM after cautiously eating half the bag of snacks slowly during the wait and the flight. My blood sugar was 122 when I arrived at the hotel. I believe food restriction based on blood glucose levels in the first few days was necessary to purge my system of excess glucose.

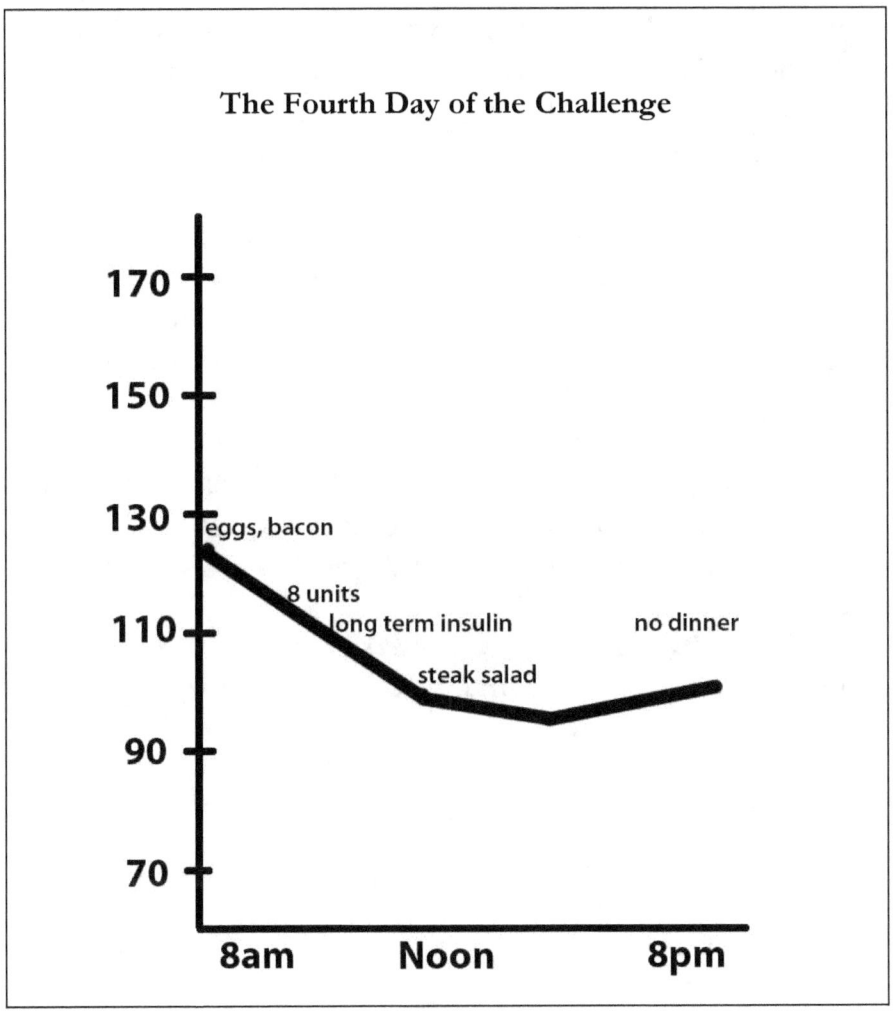

The Fourth Day of the Challenge

The following morning my sugar was about the same as the night before at 127 and I selected bacon and eggs at the hotel buffet, avoiding the waffles and bread. I took 8 units of long acting insulin. At lunchtime, my sugar was 99. At 2 PM I had a half order of a steak salad at a restaurant with relatives. At 3:30 my sugar was 94.

I skipped dinner as I had the night before. There was no food in the seasonal house anyway. At 9 PM my sugar was still 102.   I realized my body was creating sugar without any food! As a precaution I was not using insulin unless my blood sugar was above 110.   The numbers were good today but I was eating very little.

I would later learn that eggs were a good selection because the carbohydrate content is only.6 grams. Cheese also has less than a gram of carbohydrates. A bowl of unsweetened cereal, which I ate in the past, has about 25-30 grams of carbohydrates.

 I was feeling confident and motivated. It seemed like this war was going to be easy. Why couldn't everyone do this? *What was that saying? ..pride before the fall?*

I would soon learn that blood glucose levels are not only a direct result of food and insulin. Stress, infection and pain also play a role.

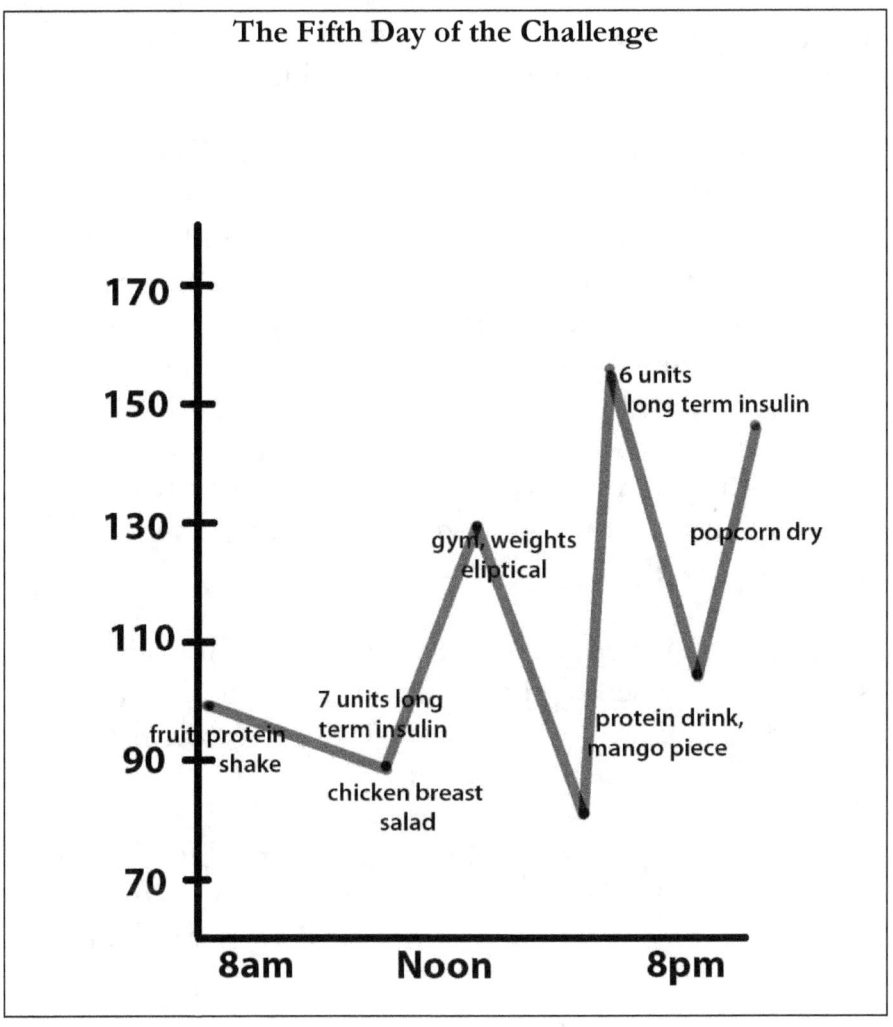

The Fifth Day of the Challenge

The following day, my sugar was 98 at 4 AM. I had a protein shake with water and a piece of mango. Near lunchtime my sugar was 89. I decided to delay my insulin until my blood sugar had risen.

At Noon I had a full chicken breast and apple pecan salad at a fast food restaurant with relatives. I followed the lunch with 7 units long acting insulin. At 1:30, my sugar was 129. I realized a full order and the added apple and sweetened pecans was too much in the salad. In spite of the insulin injection the salad increased my sugar.

I went to the gym at 4 PM worked out on weights and elliptical machine. At 5 PM, my sugar was 78 and I had a protein drink and piece of mango. Later I would learn that even a little fruit is too much for me. At 6:30 PM my sugar was 156, I took 6 units of long acting insulin. I was surprised at the dramatic increase again.

At 8:45 my sugar was 106. I felt hungry and had a snack of dry air popped popcorn. Later I would learn that popcorn always caused a spike in my sugar. At 11:45 PM my sugar was 148.

This day confirmed that I needed close monitoring. The spikes were caused by the food choices. I should have learned to always avoid popcorn and fruit. *I would still make mistakes expecting different results.*

I could not physically feel the changes in my blood sugar. I would not be able to resolve my blood sugar until I knew what it was all the time and could keep it within a normal range.

...Later I would realize that high stress usually increases my sugar by about 50 points...

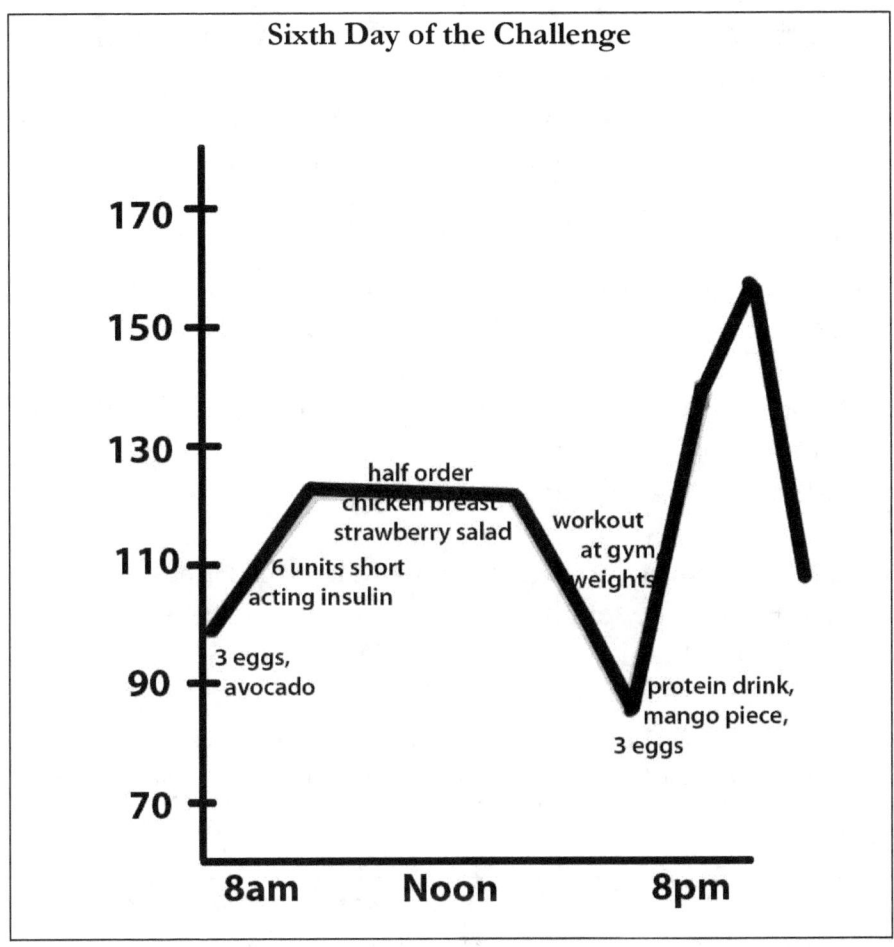

Sixth Day of the Challenge

- 170
- 150
- 130 — half order chicken breast / strawberry salad
- 110 — 6 units short acting insulin / workout at gym, weights
- 90 — 3 eggs, avocado / protein drink, mango piece, 3 eggs
- 70

8am   Noon   8pm

The following morning, my blood sugar was 101. I was impressed with my success. I believed I had enough general information to beat the sugar and was renewed in my commitment to healthy eating. Always looking for an easy answer, I thought, perhaps I would try adding short acting insulin. My prior doctor had given me short acting insulin but I was never confident about how to use it so it sat in the refrigerator. I carried it with me when I traveled.

I ate three eggs and an avocado. At 9:30 AM I tried my short acting insulin. At 10:30 AM my sugar was 123. At Noon, I had a half order of chicken breast and strawberry salad. At 2:30 my sugar was 122. At 4 PM I went to the gym and again worked out with weights and elliptical. At 4:30 my sugar was 99. At 6 PM my sugar was 86 and I drank a protein drink and ate part of a mango and three eggs. At 7 PM my sugar was 135. So far, it was working.

At 9 PM that evening I tested my glucose again and it had climbed to 153! Did my sugar normally climb all evening? I didn't know, I had never checked it so often before.

I was consistently surprised how long it takes to reduce sugar levels and how little food it takes to raise sugar levels.

Did a slice of mango affect the sugar that much? I never ate it again. Before 10:30 PM my sugar had dropped to 109.

... an entire type 2 diabetic patient population inundated with ineffective and irrelevant recommendations on websites that claim credibility...

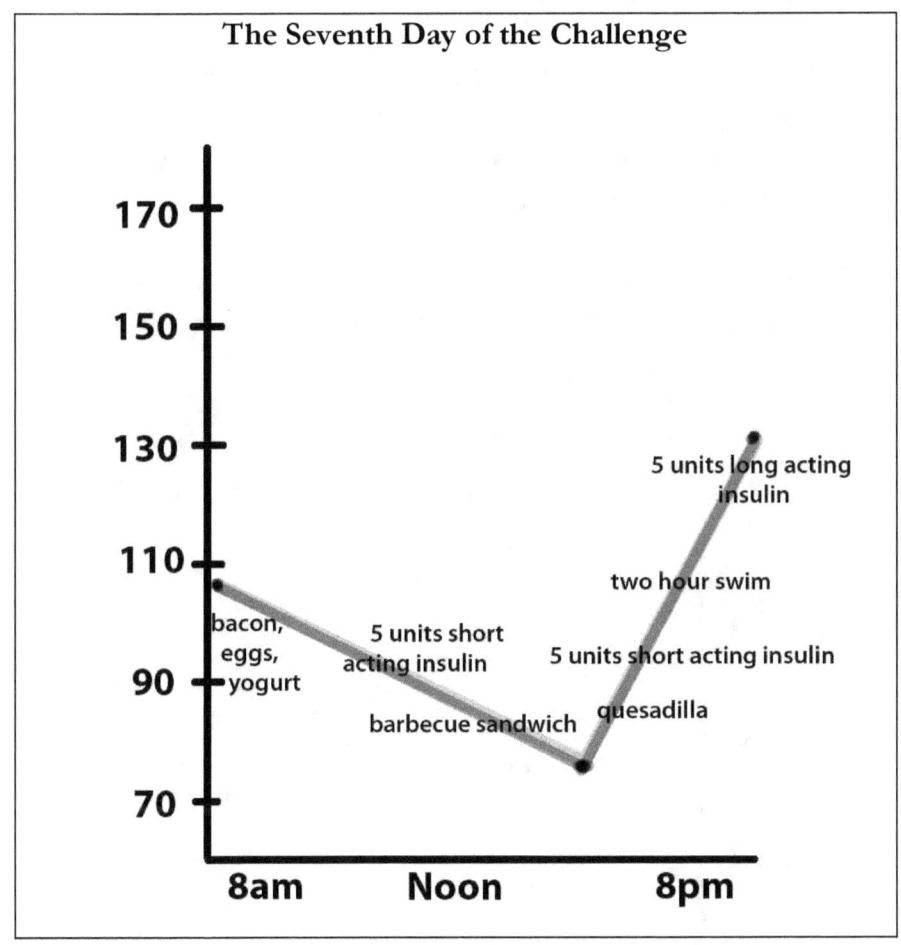

The Seventh Day of the Challenge

- bacon, eggs, yogurt
- 5 units short acting insulin
- barbecue sandwich
- quesadilla
- 5 units short acting insulin
- two hour swim
- 5 units long acting insulin

The following day, August 6, at 8 AM, I had bacon, eggs, and yogurt at the hotel buffet. At 8:30 AM I again used 5 units of the short acting insulin. At lunch I had a barbecue sandwich at the zoo with grandkids in Florida. At 5 PM my sugar was 74. I was feeling confident in my mastering of the sugar.

We ate dinner with the grandkids at the hotel restaurant. I had a quesadilla chicken and added another 5 units of short acting insulin. I swam with the kids until 10:30 PM and my sugar was still 130.

I injected 5 units of long acting insulin. I never tried the short acting insulin again because the extra and more frequent injections didn't seem to deliver any better result than the long term, especially at night.

Of course, I had barely given it a chance. I was still ignorant about insulin administration and I was callous in its use because I had never seen significant changes.

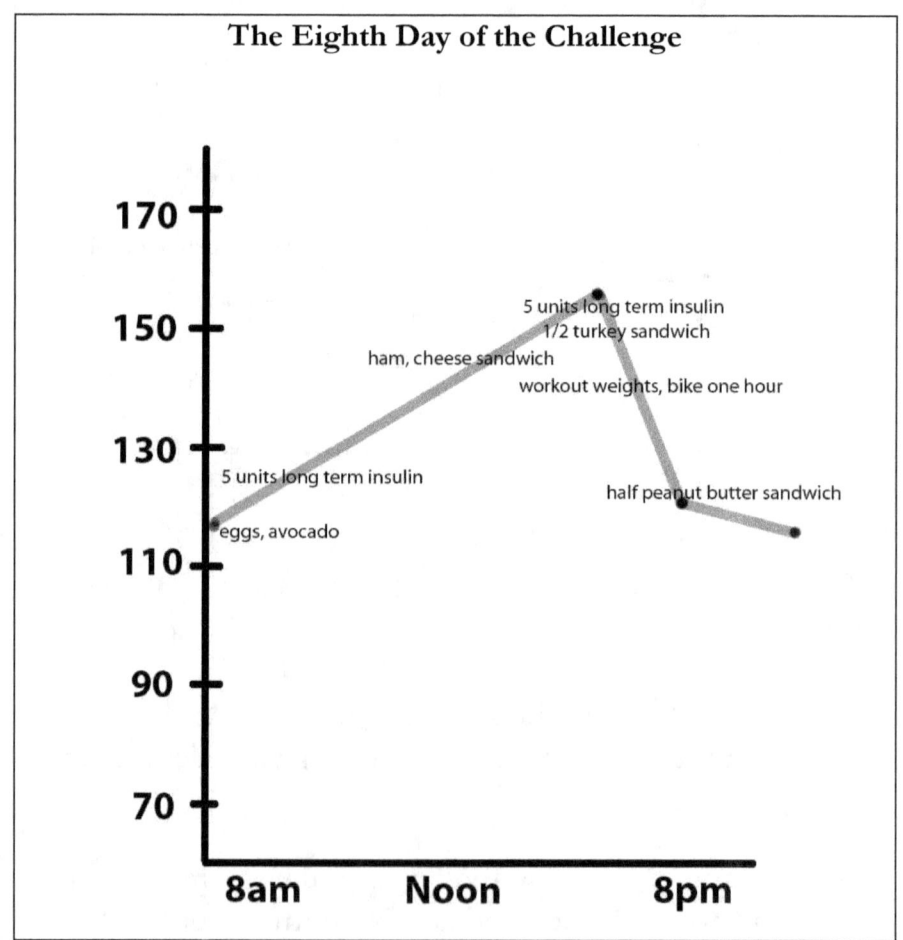

The Eighth Day of the Challenge

170

150 — 5 units long term insulin
1/2 turkey sandwich

ham, cheese sandwich

workout weights, bike one hour

130

5 units long term insulin

half peanut butter sandwich

eggs, avocado

110

90

70

8am   Noon   8pm

The following morning, I had a 115 blood sugar reading and ate eggs and avocado. An hour later I injected 5 units long acting insulin. We toured homes in central Florida and hungry at 2 PM, I ate a ham and cheese croissant sandwich at a fast food place. Later I would realize croissants had 27 carbohydrates. .

At 4 PM my sugar was 153 and I added 5 units of long acting insulin. I worked out at the hotel fitness center. The high sugar symptom pain in my neck went away after working out.

I had half a turkey sandwich at the deli. I learned quickly to limit my bread to one slice a day, later realizing it had 14 carbohydrates. My sugar was 118 and I was hungry at 9 PM. I had half a peanut butter and banana sandwich and had a sugar an hour later of 115. Later I would discover that peanut butter has 11 carbs, one slice of bread 14, and a small banana, 15.

I wanted to stop insulin because I have read that type 2 diabetes is actually resistance to insulin not a lack of insulin. I read that excess insulin promotes fat, especially around the middle.

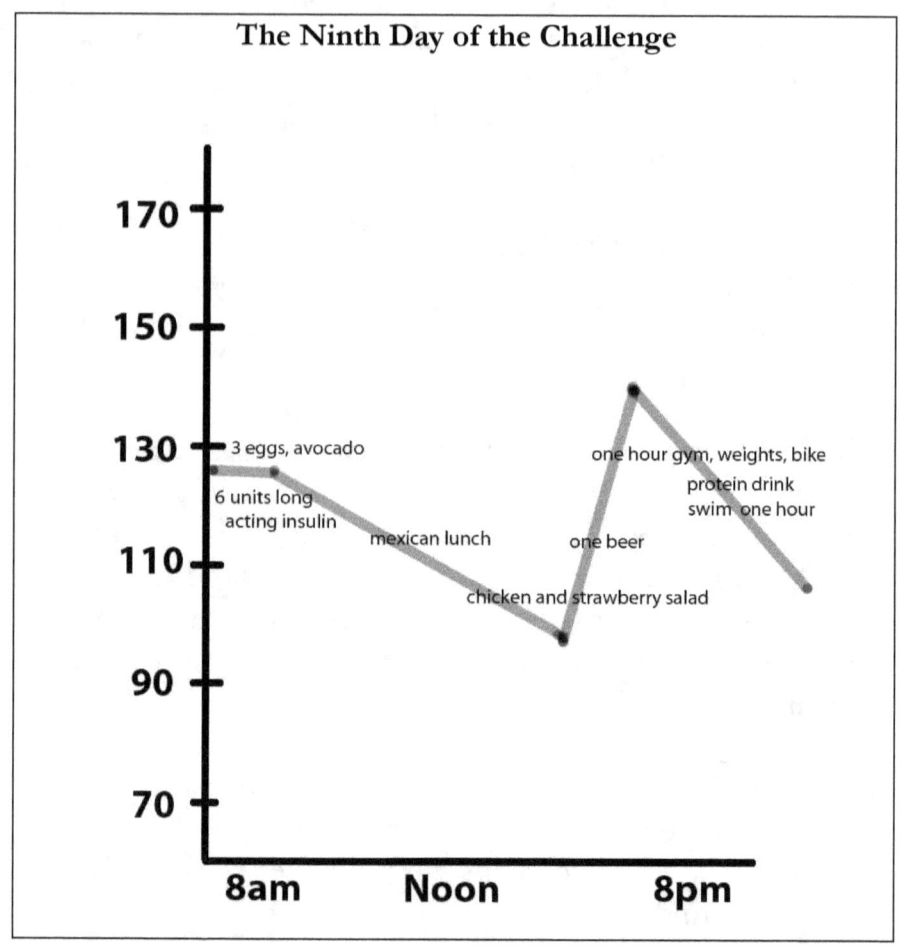

The Ninth Day of the Challenge

- 3 eggs, avocado
- 6 units long acting insulin
- mexican lunch
- chicken and strawberry salad
- one beer
- one hour gym, weights, bike
- protein drink
- swim one hour

On August 8, I again had a high fasting sugar of 128 and took 6 units of long acting insulin after eggs and avocado breakfast. At Noon we ate lunch at a local Mexican restaurant. At 4 PM after touring homes my sugar was 96. At 5 PM I ate a chicken breast and strawberry salad at a fast food restaurant.

At 6:30 PM I had one beer with my husband. At 7 PM my sugar was 140. I blamed the beer and never drank another one since. I later learned it was a good choice, beer has 13 carbs, while wine has less than 4 carbs.

I worked out with weights and the exercise bike. At 9 PM I had a protein drink. I swam with grandkids until 11 PM when my sugar was 107. **I realized the gym weight workouts had the same or better effect in the evening as the long term insulin.** Weights also had a better impact than my long bike rides.

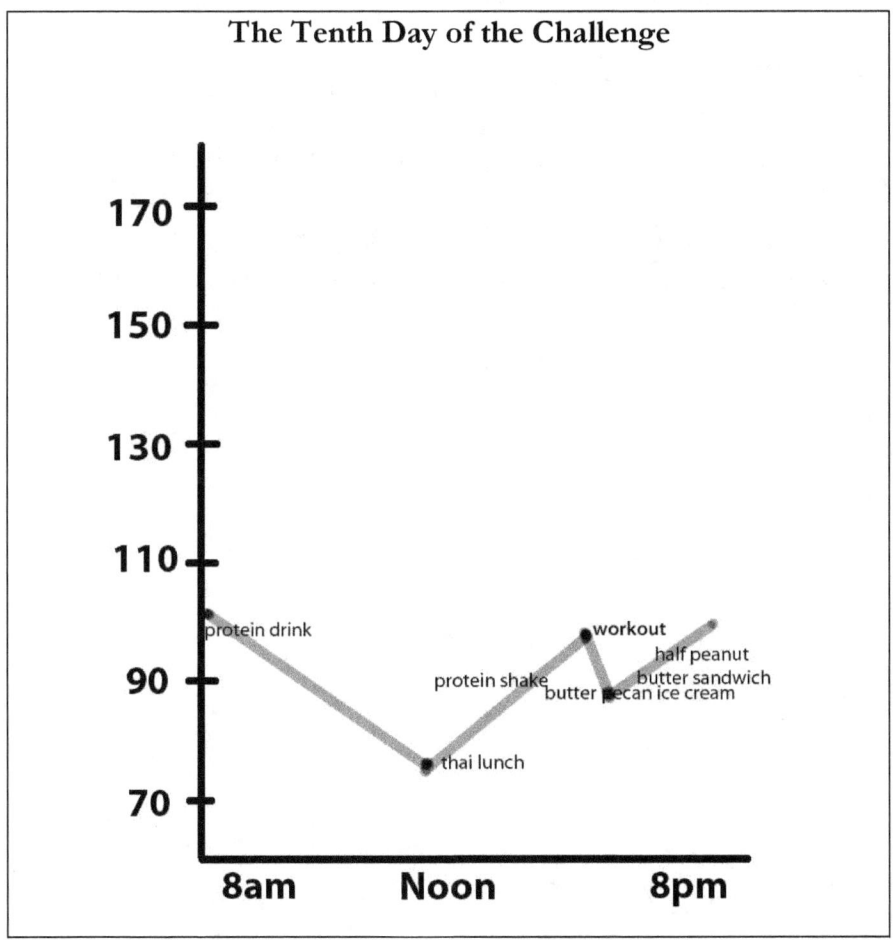

Breakthrough #1   After Ten Days Finally!

August 9 was a breakthrough day. I woke with a sugar of 106. I had a protein drink and at 11:30 AM, a 75 sugar. I had a Thai lunch, soup, salad, sesame noodle entree, pork satay and at 4 PM my sugar was 100. At 4:30 PM I had a protein shake and at 5 PM worked out with weights in the gym. After the workout, I had a scoop of butter pecan ice cream and had a 90 blood sugar immediately afterward. *Have I healed my pancreas already?*

At 6 PM I was hungry and ate a half peanut butter sandwich. At 9 PM I had a 100 blood sugar. I never took insulin all day and blood sugars remained stable.

...Curiously, in the early morning my fasting sugar can have dramatic changes over a couple hours without any food or drink...

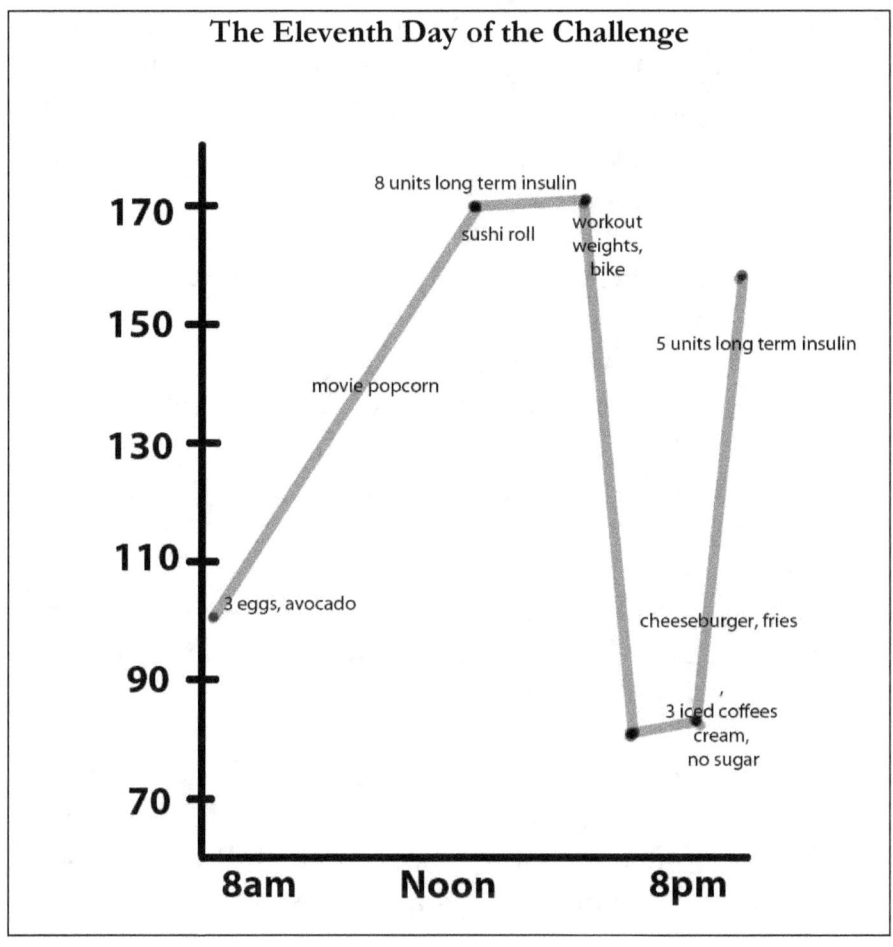

The Eleventh Day of the Challenge

8 units long term insulin
sushi roll
workout weights, bike
5 units long term insulin
movie popcorn
3 eggs, avocado
cheeseburger, fries
3 iced coffees cream, no sugar

170
150
130
110
90
70

8am   Noon   8pm

On August 10, at 7 AM I had a 106 blood sugar and ate three eggs and an avocado. I remember reading once that avocado is the perfect fat to eat with an egg. Later I would discover that at 14 grams of carbohydrate, it is one of the better fruit choices. My husband and I went to a movie matinee and ate dry popcorn. Months later I would learn that a large popcorn has 26 grams of carbohydrates. I was feeling overly confident with my blood sugars after yesterday. Today would be a new learning experience.

After the movie I had a 170 blood sugar! I injected 8 units long acting insulin. I could feel the familiar high blood sugar symptoms in the back of my neck. I shared a sushi roll lunch with my husband who was hungry, and at 4 PM I still had a 171 blood sugar.

I had not learned yet how high white rice was in carbohydrates. A cup of rice has 50 grams of carbohydrate, higher than bread, and more than a slice of chocolate cake. I have learned to avoid Asian and Mexican meals with their rice components. Rice is worse than potatoes. It is promoted as a healthy food choice in many diets.

At 5 PM I worked out with weights, elliptical and bike and at 5:30 had an 84 blood sugar. I indulged in my favorite treat, iced coffees with cream.

At 9 PM I had a dinner of cheeseburger and fries with grandkids at the hotel. It was an unusual meal for me but there were limited options. *Yikes*, at 10:30 PM I had 163 sugar and took 5 units of long acting insulin.

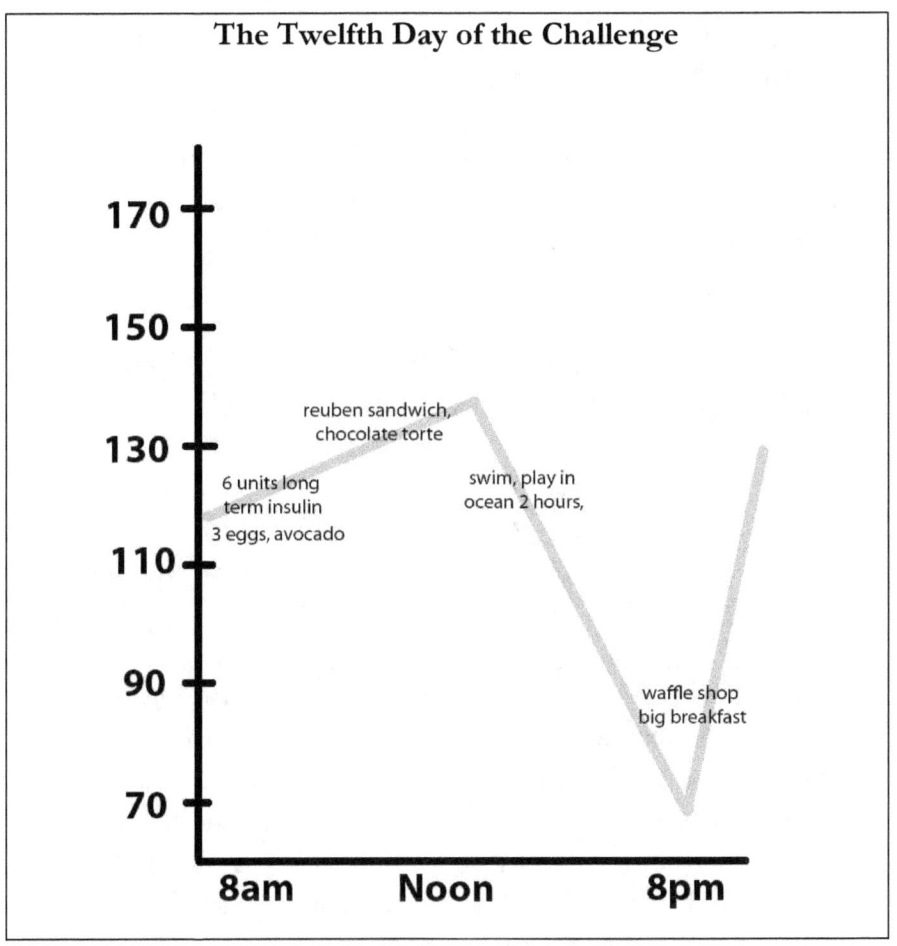

The Twelfth Day of the Challenge

170
150
130 — reuben sandwich, chocolate torte
6 units long term insulin
3 eggs, avocado
110 — swim, play in ocean 2 hours,
90 — waffle shop big breakfast
70

8am   Noon   8pm

Breakthrough #2 Low Sugar Days In Spite of Sandwich Meals

On August 11, at 7 AM I had a 118 blood sugar. I was relieved it had dropped significantly since last night. I took 6 units of long acting insulin. At 8 AM, I had three eggs and an avocado. At lunch, I had a reuben sandwich and chocolate torte dessert with relatives in a Cocoa Beach restaurant. Corned beef I discovered later has only 1/3 gram of carbohydrate, swiss cheese ½ gram and pumpernickel bread 12 grams per slice. The chocolate torte probably contained about 40 grams.

I swam with the grandkids at the pool and in the ocean for two hours. At 8 PM my sugar was 70 and I was seriously hungry. It was the first time I felt hunger with low blood sugar for a long time.

Previously when I had been hungry my blood sugar was actually high. We ate dinner at 9 PM at a waffle shop, a big breakfast.

I realized I could not tell from my symptoms whether I was hungry due to low or high blood sugar. Sometimes when craving food my blood sugar was actually high, not low.

I read that symptoms of too low sugar are hunger, sweating, restlessness, speech impairment, confusion, tremor, difficulty concentrating, drowsiness, headache, and visual disturbances. I never felt these effects, but I had a friend on an insulin pump who experienced this while at my home. It took several cookies and glucose tablets and at least an hour to increase his sugar.

Below 70 blood sugar is considered hypoglycemic and under 50 can cause insulin shock.

I discovered that when I have difficulty sleeping or wake up with a fast heartbeat my sugar is often high. Perhaps it is the result of stress or late snacking. High sugar does impact sleep quality.

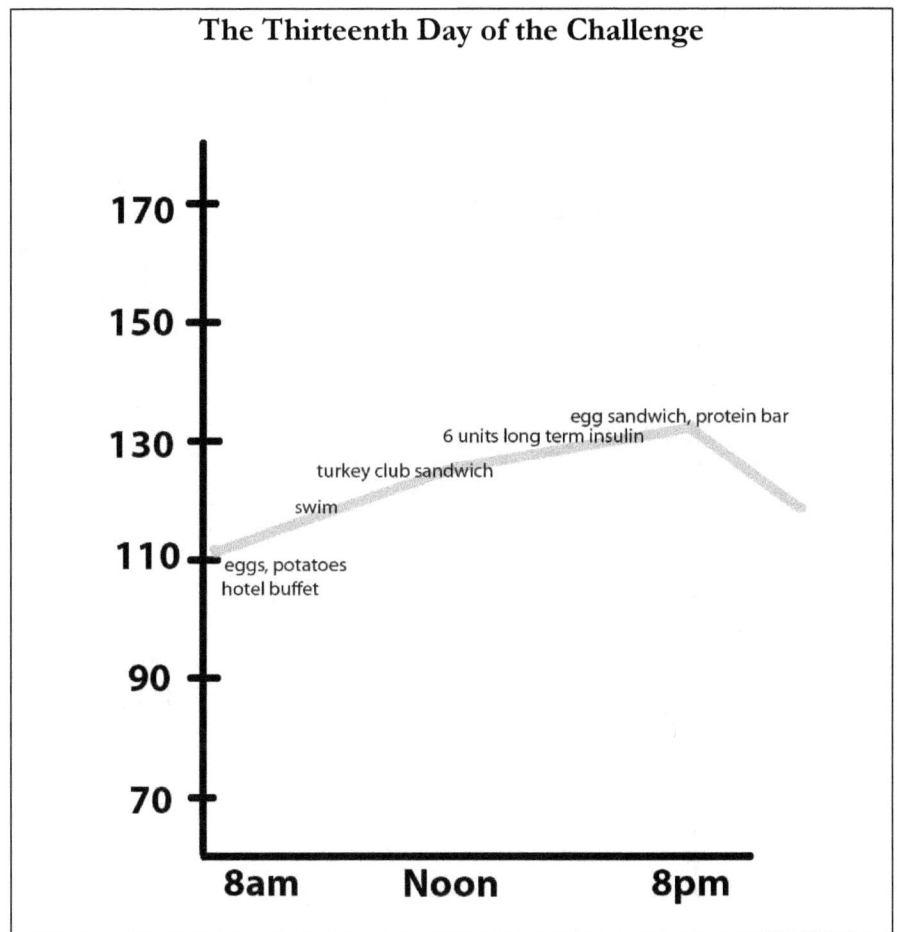

The Thirteenth Day of the Challenge

170

150

130 — egg sandwich, protein bar
6 units long term insulin

turkey club sandwich

swim

110 — eggs, potatoes
hotel buffet

90

70

8am   Noon   8pm

On August 12, at 7 AM, I had a blood sugar of 110. I ate eggs and potatoes at the hotel buffet breakfast. At Noon my blood sugar was 128. I hadn't taken insulin in the morning because my blood sugar was not over 110. I took 6 units of long acting insulin after lunch.

At 1 PM we ate a turkey sandwich at the airport. Six hours later in Illinois, at 7 PM, I had a breakfast egg sandwich and a protein bar. At 10 PM my blood sugar was 120. It was a relatively good day.

I still haven't lost any weight but I am hoping that will occur. I feel more energy with the lower sugar levels.

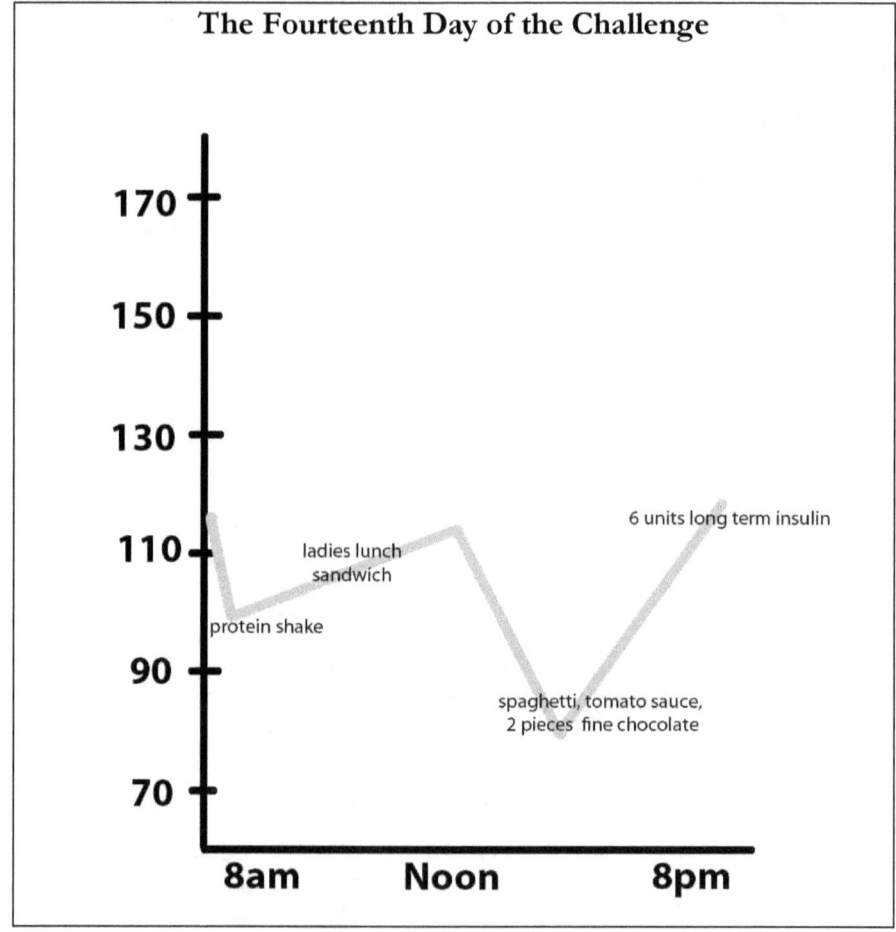

The Fourteenth Day of the Challenge

170
150
130
110 — ladies lunch sandwich
protein shake
6 units long term insulin
90 — spaghetti, tomato sauce, 2 pieces fine chocolate
70

8am   Noon   8pm

On August 13, at 6 AM my sugar was 115, it dropped further and at 8 AM, 106. **Curiously, in the early morning my fasting sugar can have dramatic changes**

over a couple hours without any food or drink. I drank a protein shake at 8 AM. At Noon I met a friend for lunch. At 5 PM my blood sugar was 78. At 6 PM I served spaghetti sauce and pasta and two pieces of gourmet chocolate. Later I discovered pasta noodles have 19 grams of carbs for ½ cup and the pasta sauce has about 13. At 8:30 PM my sugar was 126 and I injected 6 units long acting insulin. It was another successful day but my challenges would not be over.

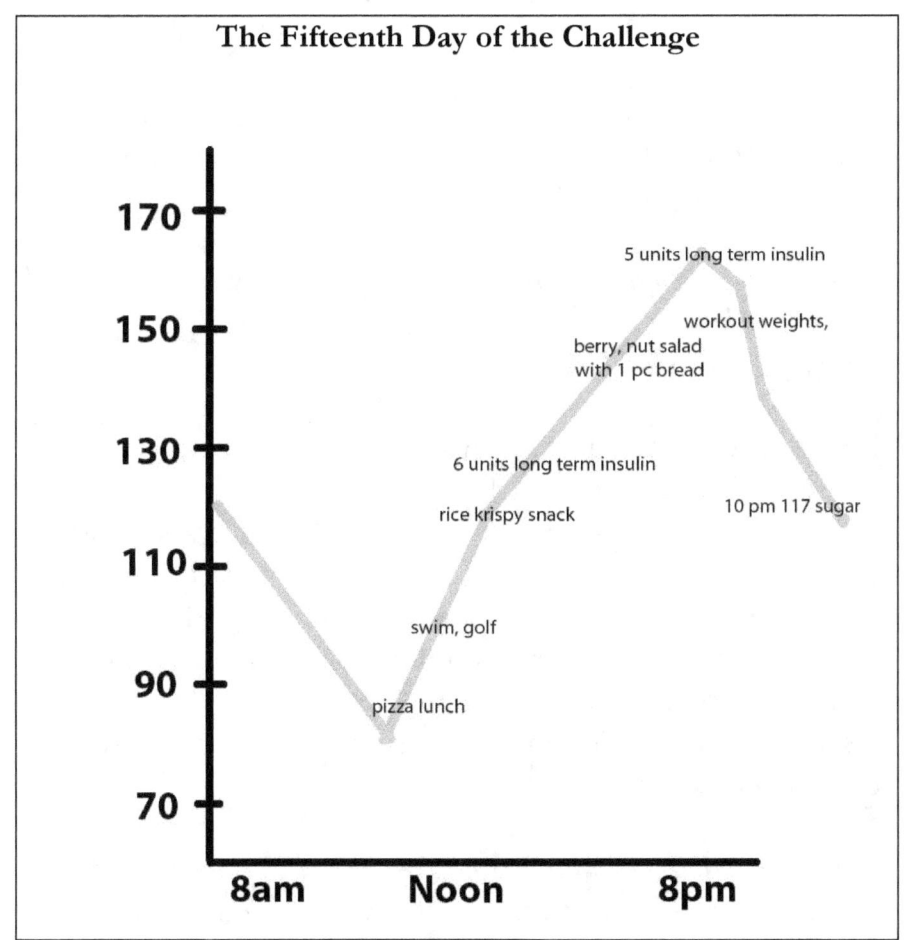

The Fifteenth Day of the Challenge

- 170
- 150 — 5 units long term insulin
- workout weights, berry, nut salad with 1 pc bread
- 130 — 6 units long term insulin
- rice krispy snack
- 10 pm 117 sugar
- 110
- swim, golf
- 90 — pizza lunch
- 70

8am   Noon   8pm

On August 14, my blood sugar was 120 when I woke. I skipped breakfast. At Noon, my sugar was 78. We shared a pizza with our grandkids. I played golf and swam with a friend during the afternoon and at 5 PM after a treat, my sugar was 120. I injected 6 units of long acting insulin and we met friends at a local restaurant for a favorite large berry nut salad entree with warm bread. Since this meal I have never had fruit or accompanied my salad with bread

My sugar was 166 two hours later! I injected another 5 units long acting insulin. Again I wondered if the insulin was working.

At 8:30 PM I lifted weights and at 9 PM my sugar was 138, at 10 PM, it was 117.

Bread, rice and potatoes were the sugar producers for me. Boiled and mashed cauliflower was my substitute for potatoes until the craving subsided for a starchy side.

I have recently begun to monitor the carbohydrate content of soups. The carbohydrate content is usually listed for 2.5 servings per can. Chicken noodle soup has 8 grams of carbs and split pea, 26 grams. I used to wonder why a can of tomato soup caused me to be sleepy after eating. Now I realize some contain high fructose corn syrup. Soups in restaurants have been off my diet since I discovered my reaction to monosodium glutamate, MSG, or hydrolyzed protein years ago.

...In recent months I realized that many vegetable components of fresh salads are high in carbohydrates. I have found I can only tolerate small portions of fresh salads. Salads are not the free food

that I formerly believed. dressings and fruit pieces are especially high in carbohydrates...

I recently have found a wide range of carbohydrates on bread labels. Pita and croissants are particularly bad, at 33 and 27 grams. Whole grain breads are only 2 grams less than white bread and yet are promoted as a healthy option.

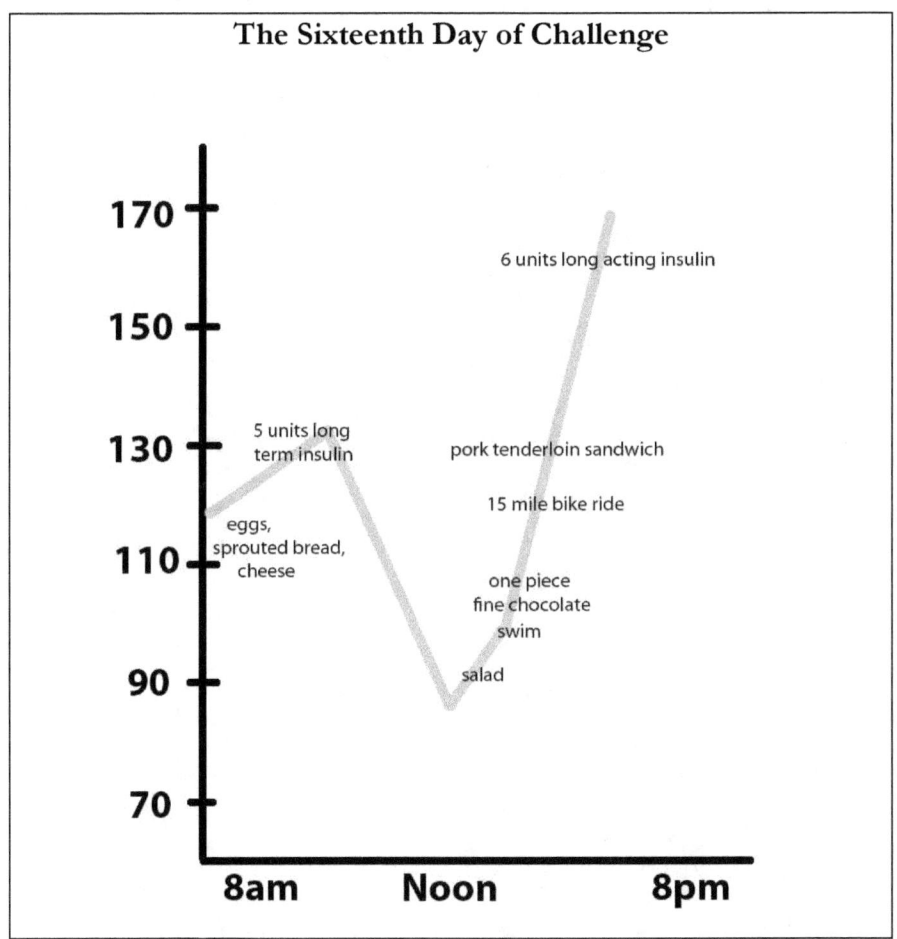

The Sixteenth Day of Challenge

170

150

130 — 5 units long term insulin — pork tenderloin sandwich

15 mile bike ride

110 — eggs, sprouted bread, cheese

one piece fine chocolate

swim

90 — salad

70

8am   Noon   8pm

6 units long acting insulin

I woke at 6 AM with 117 sugar. I had eggs and cheese on sprouted bread and injected 5 units long acting insulin. At Noon my sugar was 87 and I had a salad lunch. At 2 PM I swam and had one piece of gourmet chocolate. At 3 PM I had 99 sugar. At 4 PM I went on a 15 mile bike ride and ate a pork tenderloin, without the bun, and diet coke.

At 6:30 PM I had a sugar of 167! I injected 6 units long acting insulin. This challenge has not been won yet. I did not feel I had overeaten today. *Why is my sugar so high? Do I have pain, infection or stress?*

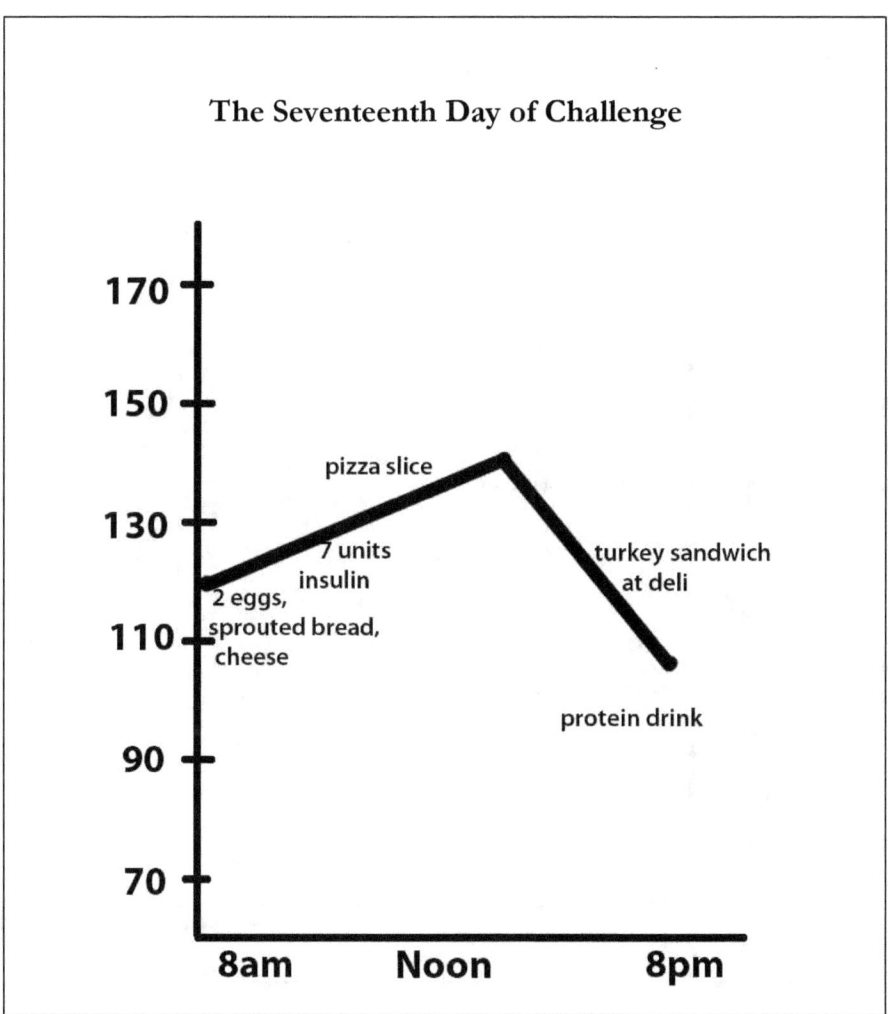

The Seventeenth Day of Challenge

pizza slice

7 units
insulin

2 eggs,
sprouted bread,
cheese

turkey sandwich
at deli

protein drink

170 150 130 110 90 70

8am   Noon   8pm

My sugar dropped during the night. I woke with 120 sugar and injected 7 units long acting insulin. I ate two eggs, sprouted bread and cheese. At Noon we shared two pizza slices. At 2 PM, I had 141 sugar. At 4 PM we drove to

Wisconsin and stopped at a deli for a turkey sandwich. At 7 PM my sugar was 105 and I had a protein drink.

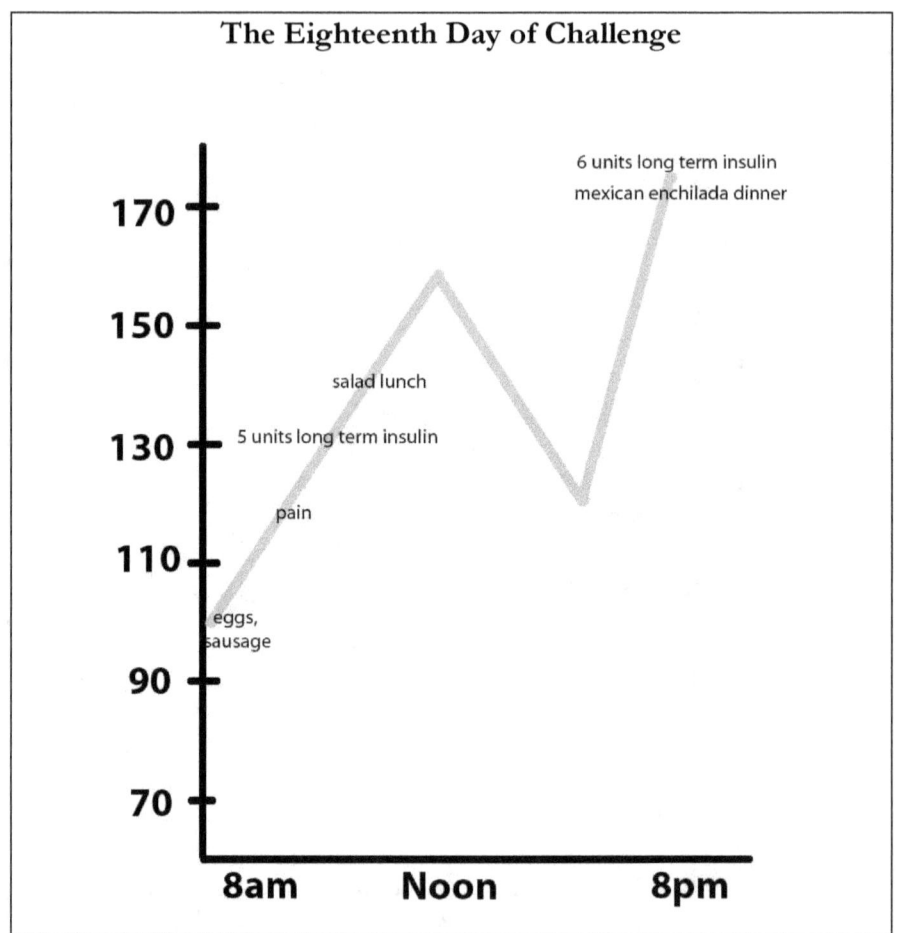

The Eighteenth Day of Challenge

6 units long term insulin
mexican enchilada dinner

salad lunch

5 units long term insulin

pain

eggs,
sausage

170
150
130
110
90
70

8am   Noon   8pm

I woke with 104 blood sugar. I had eggs, sausage, and my sugar began to rise and at 9 AM I injected 5 units of insulin. It measured 161 after salad lunch. I felt the familiar signs of high blood sugar in the back of my neck that ached. It would get worse, Mexican food was one of the worst options for dinner. I did not care at the moment.

Was it stress, pain or infection? It doesn't seem to be due to my diet today. I did record pain in my notes. The sugar is on a dramatic rise throughout the day in spite of reasonable choices for breakfast and lunch.

According to some researchers more pancreatic beta cells are destroyed each time the blood sugar spikes. One study found a 4 day exposure to elevated glucose could cause the damage. The worse the spike, the faster damage is created.

One of the habits I picked up from my husband was adding yogurt after meals. A 6 ounce fruit flavored yogurt cup has about 20 grams of carbohydrates. I have stopped eating yogurt entirely.

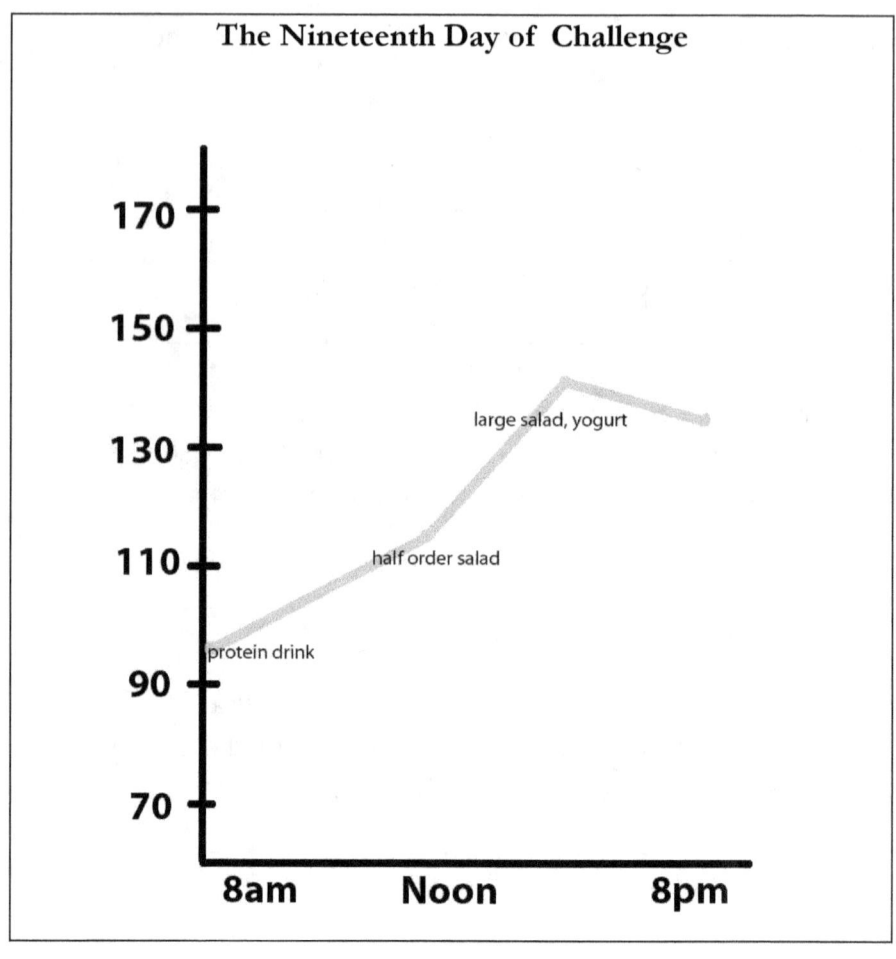

The Nineteenth Day of Challenge

170
150
130
large salad, yogurt
110
half order salad
protein drink
90
70

8am   Noon   8pm

On day 19 I woke with 96 blood sugar. It was a relief after the day before. I would be more careful today. I had a half order Chicken Breast salad for lunch. My blood sugar was 116 at 2 PM. I had no insulin in the morning because my blood sugar was below 110.

At 6 PM I made a large dinner salad with cheese, lunch meat, nuts. I had learned to avoid the fruit and many vegetables in my salads. Meal planning would have been so much easier if I had remembered the total carbohydrate connection to glucose. At 7:30 PM my sugar was 143. I had added a small yogurt after the salad meal. *Was the yogurt to blame? I never ate yogurt again.*

At 8:30 PM my blood sugar was 133. Tomorrow would be even worse.

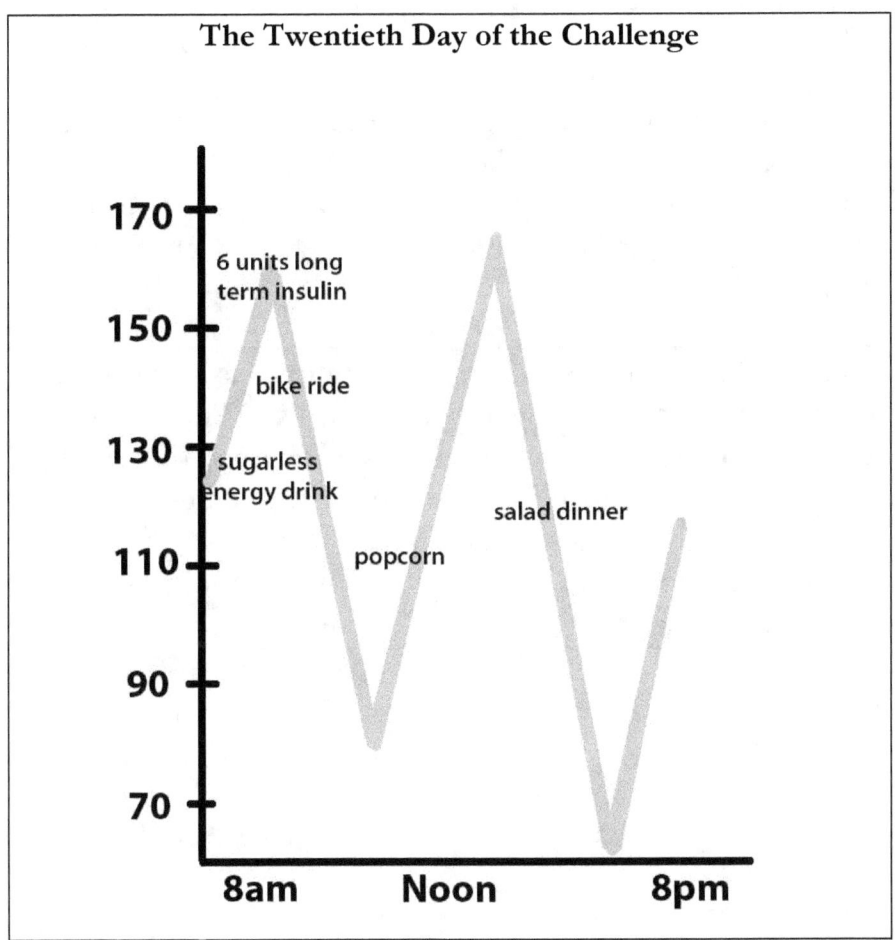

The Twentieth Day of the Challenge

- 6 units long term insulin
- bike ride
- sugarless energy drink
- popcorn
- salad dinner

170 / 150 / 130 / 110 / 90 / 70

8am — Noon — 8pm

On August 19, I had a protein and a sugarless fruit energy drink and then measured 157 blood sugar. Was it the fruit energy drink again? *Didn't my system realize it was sugarless?* I took 6 units long acting insulin. We did a 15 mile bike ride and before Noon I had a blood sugar of 83. We went to a movie at lunchtime and I tried popcorn again. *Yes, I am a slow learner and very stubborn!*

At 4 PM my sugar was 167. I made a large salad dinner and at 7:30 had a 66 sugar. Apparently my system had a delayed response to the high sugar from the popcorn. These swings are very bad. At 7:30 PM it returned to 116.

This was not a good day. It is harmful to beta cells in my pancreas to have high spikes in glucose levels. *Was this the dramatic swing in glucose my doctor warned me about?* I realized if I wanted to quit the insulin I must get control of my diet.

When we travel I now rely on cashew nuts as a snack. 20 cashews have about 5 carbohydrates only. When we must eat out at fast food restaurants, I choose 4 chicken nuggets without sauce because it has had the best outcome on my sugar levels. Later I would learn that the carbohydrate content of 6 nuggets is about the same as one slice of bread.

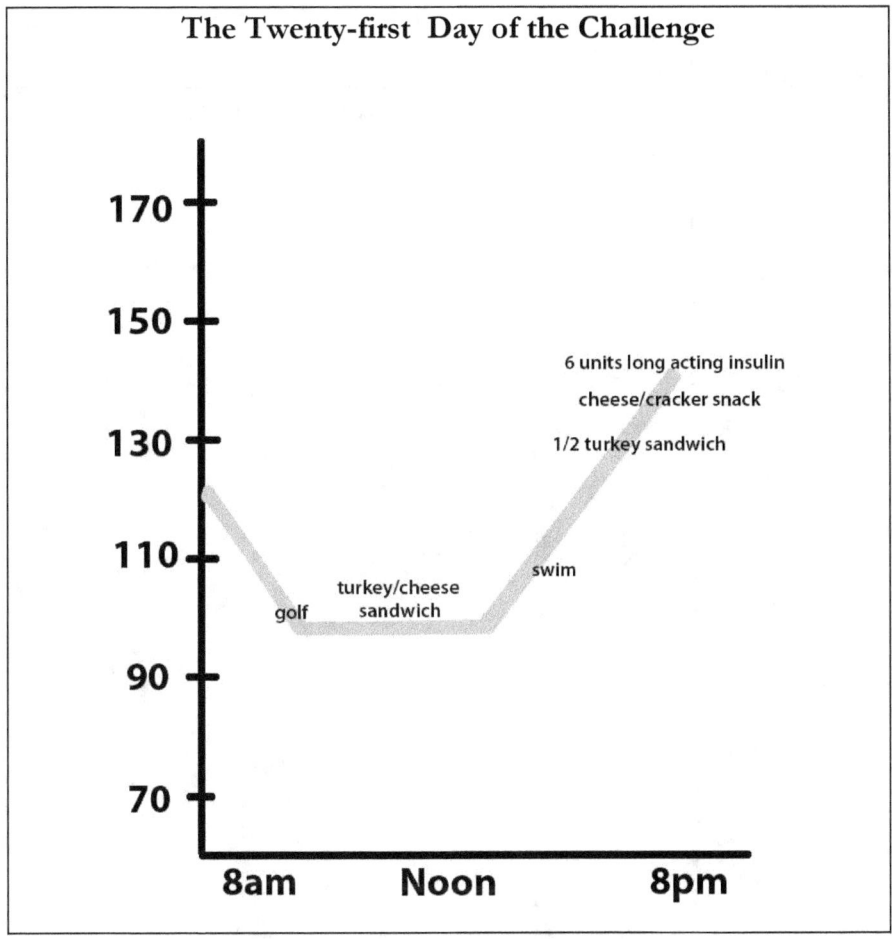

The Twenty-first Day of the Challenge

170

150

130

110

90

70

6 units long acting insulin

cheese/cracker snack

1/2 turkey sandwich

swim

turkey/cheese sandwich

golf

8am   Noon   8pm

On August 20 I woke with 117 sugar. At 10:30 AM it was 103. I played an hour of golf with a friend. At Noon we had a turkey and cheese sandwich on pumpernickel bread. At 3:30 my sugar was 105. We swam for two hours. At 8:30 PM I had a half turkey sandwich. I ate a few cheese and cracker snacks. Later I would realize the butter crackers had 50 grams of carbohydrates. At 10 PM I had a blood sugar 145! I injected 6 units long acting insulin. It was the first dose of insulin all day. *Could an evening snack have this much impact?*

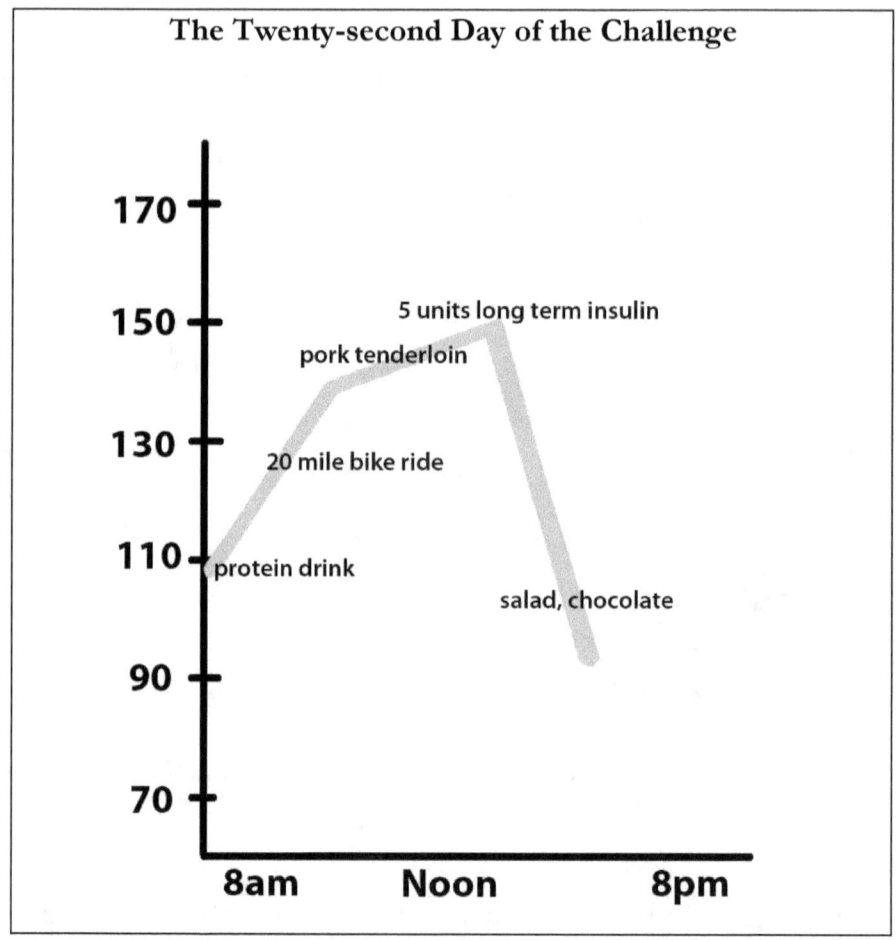

The Twenty-second Day of the Challenge

170

150 — 5 units long term insulin

pork tenderloin

130

20 mile bike ride

110 — protein drink

salad, chocolate

90

70

8am   Noon   8pm

On August 21, I woke with 110 sugar and had a protein drink. At 10:30 AM it was 138. At 11 AM I did a 20 mile bike ride and at 1 PM had a pork tenderloin. At 2:30 PM I had 150 sugar. Frustrated at the persistent sugar, at 3 PM I injected 5 units long acting insulin. At 4:30 PM I had 92 sugar. *That is better!* At 6 PM I made a large salad dinner with a piece of chocolate.

I discovered that emotional stress impacted my sugar levels regardless of what I had eaten. I found that appointments with an attorney resulted in 50 point increases in post meal sugar levels. I also experienced 50 point increases in post meal sugar levels when I babysat for preschool grandchildren. In my current diary I started noting high stress days which I had not done previously.

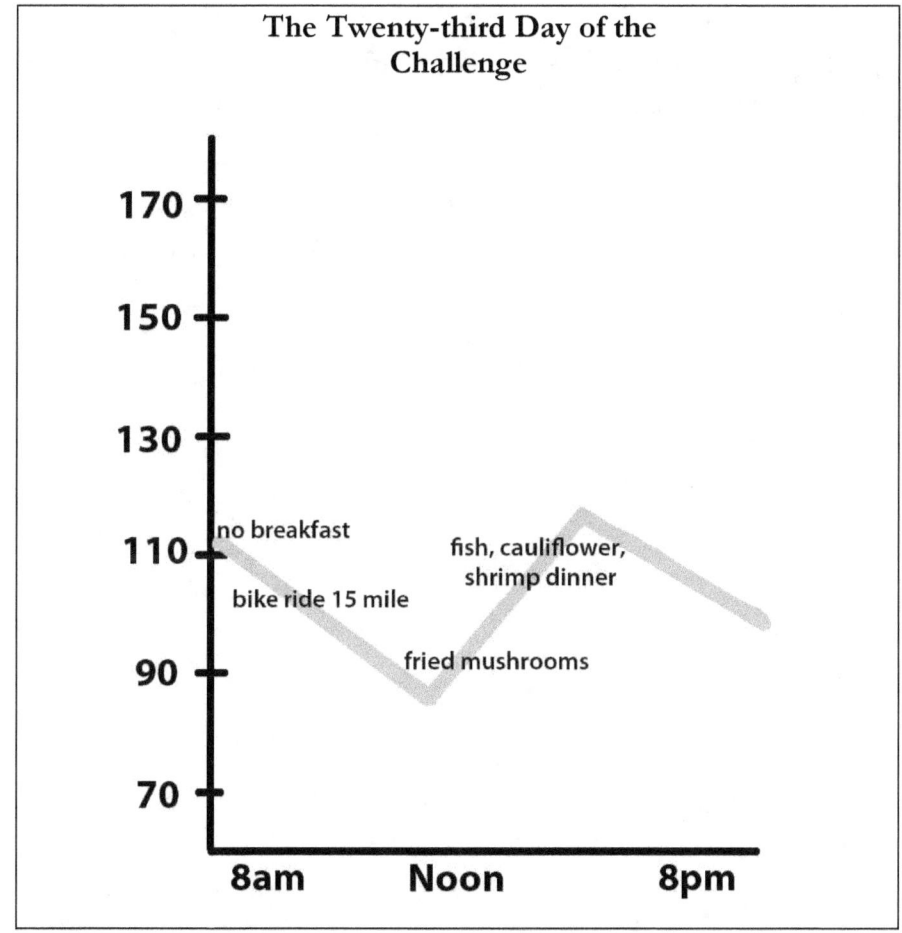

The Twenty-third Day of the Challenge

170
150
130
110   no breakfast
      bike ride 15 mile
90   fried mushrooms
70

fish, cauliflower, shrimp dinner

8am   Noon   8pm

On August 22 I woke with 110 sugar. I was no longer as afraid of low blood sugars so I skipped breakfast. I did a

15 mike bike ride and ate breaded mushrooms. At 12:30 PM I had an 88 sugar.

At 6 PM I hosted a neighbor for dinner, I served fish baked with shrimp soup sauce, creamed cauliflower, and green beans with red wine. At 8 PM my sugar was 113. At 3 AM it was 99.

This was a good day without the spikes and troughs perhaps because or in spite of no insulin. This was the second time I had a good day after avoiding breakfast. *Perhaps a coincidence?*

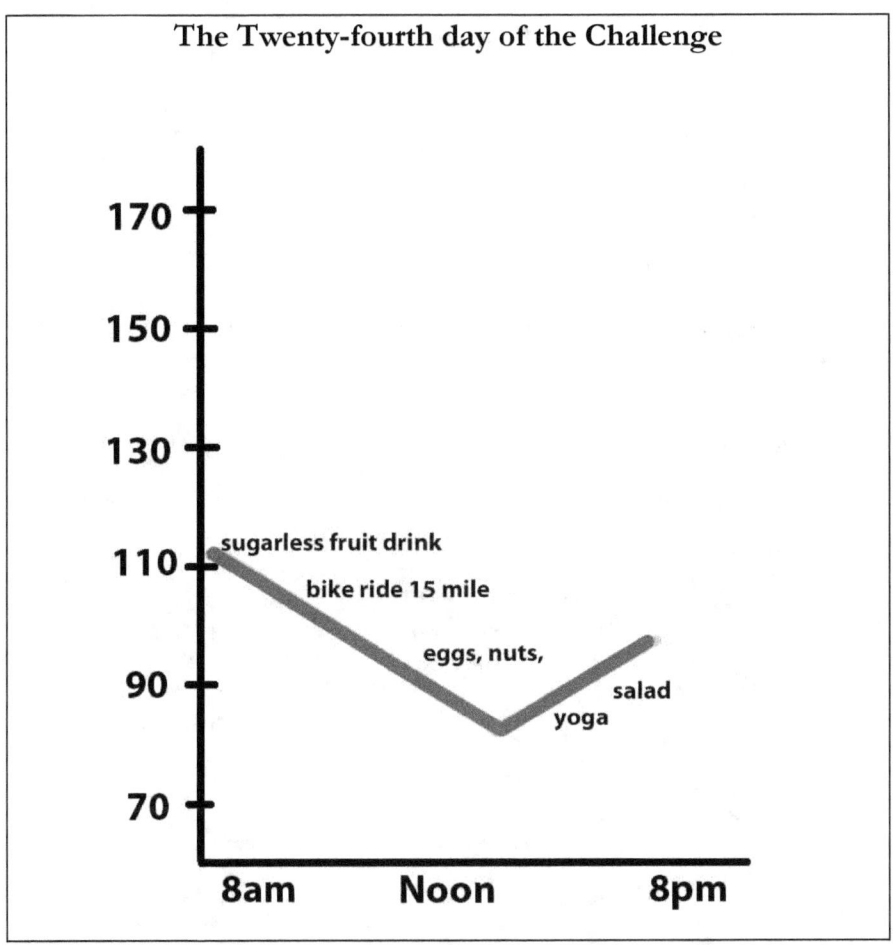

The Twenty-fourth day of the Challenge

On August 23, I woke with 112 sugar. I had the sugarless drink and today it did not result in excessive sugar. For lunch I ate eggs and nuts after a bike ride. I had a salad for dinner. I was getting a bit smarter about ingredients. No insulin today, and another good day.

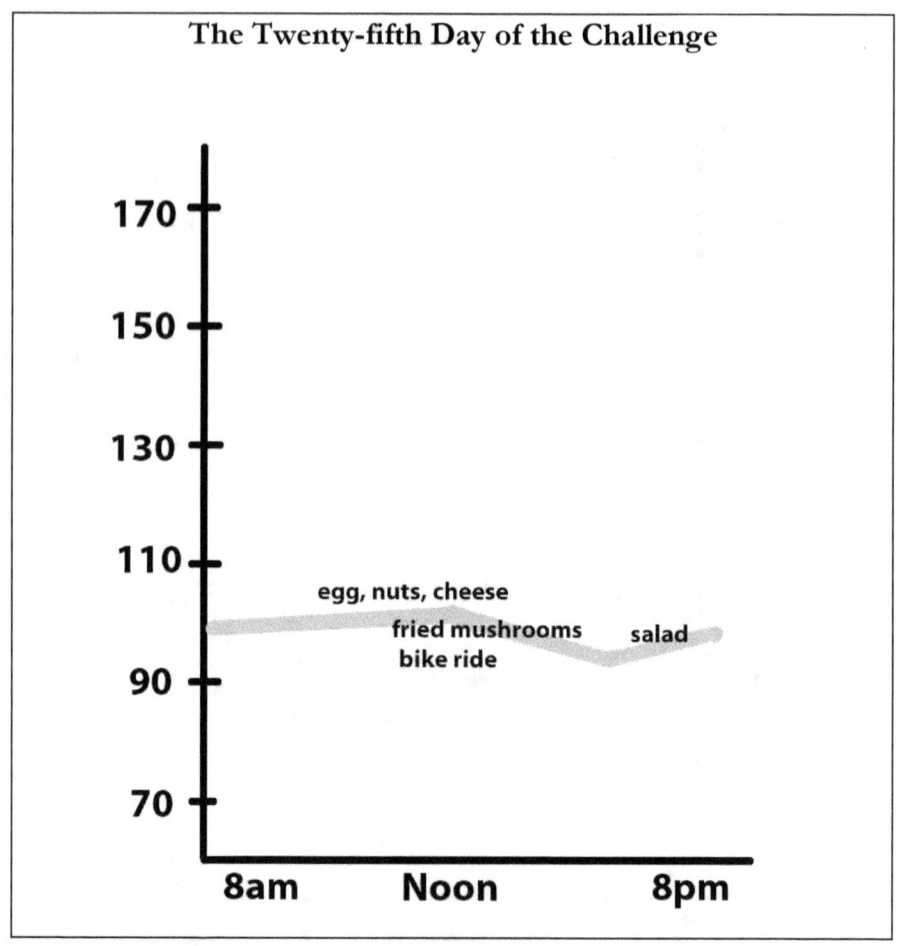

The Twenty-fifth Day of the Challenge

170
150
130
110

egg, nuts, cheese
fried mushrooms   salad
bike ride

90
70

8am   Noon   8pm

On August 24, I woke with 101 sugar and at Noon a 103 sugar. For lunch I had egg, nuts, cheese. At 1 PM I did a 15 mile bike ride and ate fried mushrooms. At 5 PM my sugar was 105 and at 6 PM I served a large salad dinner. At 7:30 PM my sugar was 107. No insulin today and again, no spikes or troughs. It is as if I am non diabetic! This may be the victory. *Is it all about skipping breakfast?*

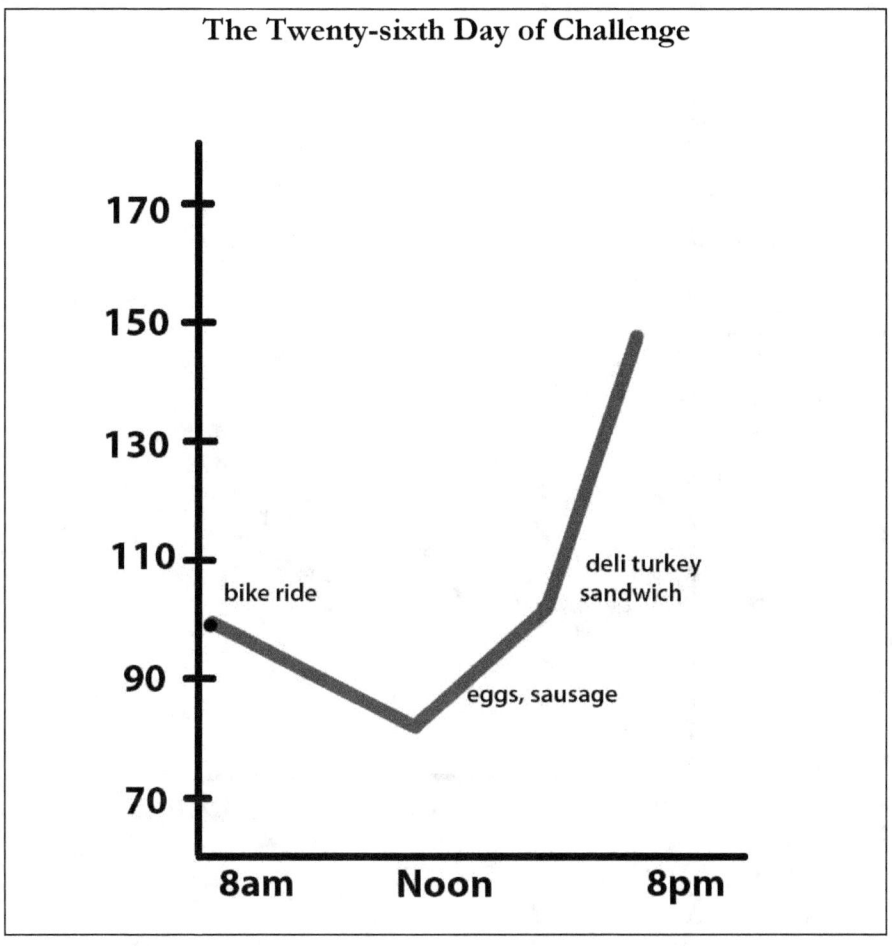

The Twenty-sixth Day of Challenge

bike ride

eggs, sausage

deli turkey sandwich

170
150
130
110
90
70

8am   Noon   8pm

Today was not as good as yesterday. I was reluctant to go back to insulin. Even with a restricted diet, and no breakfast, in the evening the blood sugar rose significantly. The deli turkey sandwich had not affected my sugar this much in the past. *Perhaps it is stress on the drive to Wisconsin?* Sometimes it is more than food or insulin, it is stress, pain or infection.

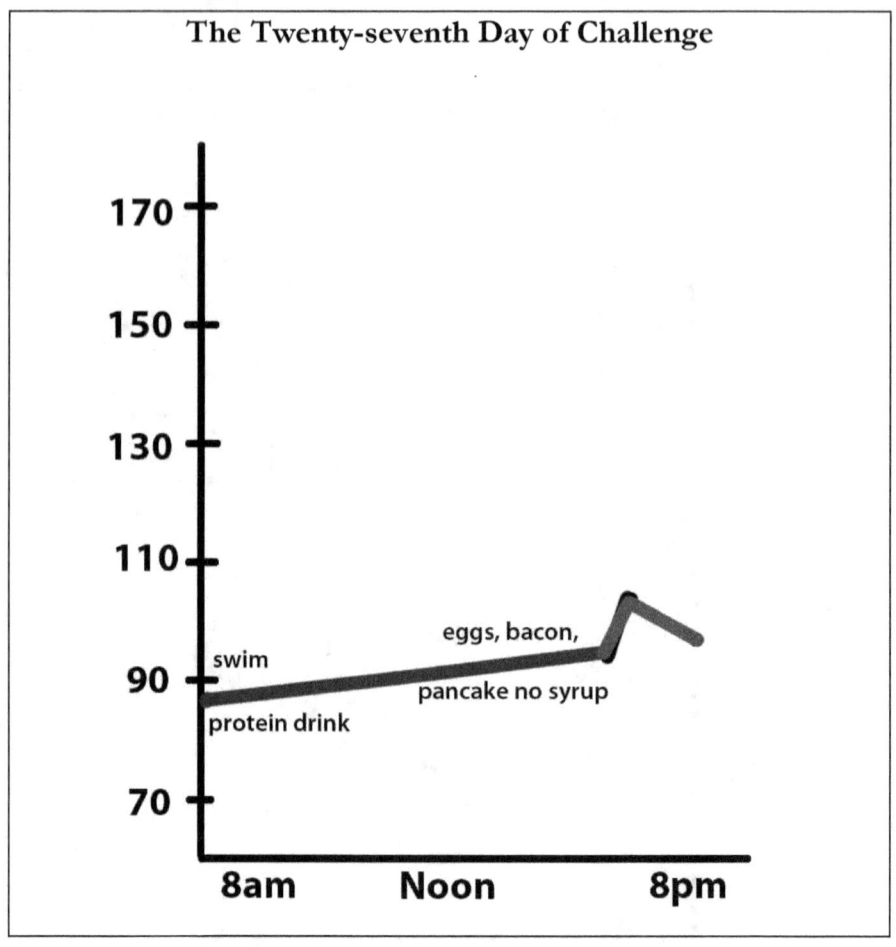

The Twenty-seventh Day of Challenge

170
150
130
110
90
70

eggs, bacon,
swim
pancake no syrup
protein drink

8am   Noon   8pm

On the twenty-seventh day I had consistently low sugar without insulin. I could observe changes in my ability to tolerate glucose. In the first days of the challenge I could not have eaten pancakes even without syrup.

I have read that peak blood sugar occurs at 45 minutes after eating a meal and sugar returns to normal five hours later. I believe my sugar levels remained high much longer.

It was difficult to find cause and effect when prior meals were still creating highs. It was important for me not to eat soon after a previous meal. I had to wait until my blood sugar dropped before eating again. I violated my own rule many times to avoid eating until my blood glucose was below 110. The negative result can be clearly demonstrated on my challenge.

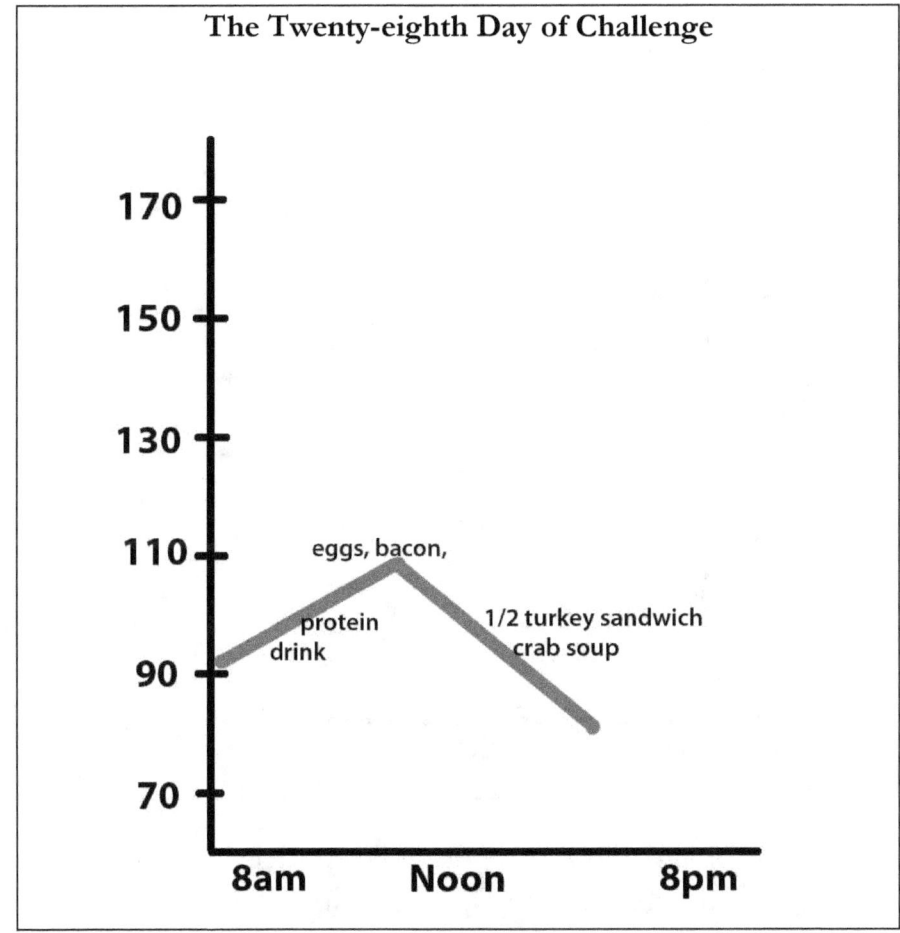

The Twenty-eighth Day of Challenge

170
150
130
110 — eggs, bacon,
protein
drink — 1/2 turkey sandwich
crab soup
90
70

8am   Noon   8pm

On the 28th day I continued the downtrend in the glucose spikes in spite of no insulin. I am still relying on breakfast foods, eggs and meat. On this day I ate breakfast food for lunch. It seems better to delay my first meal.

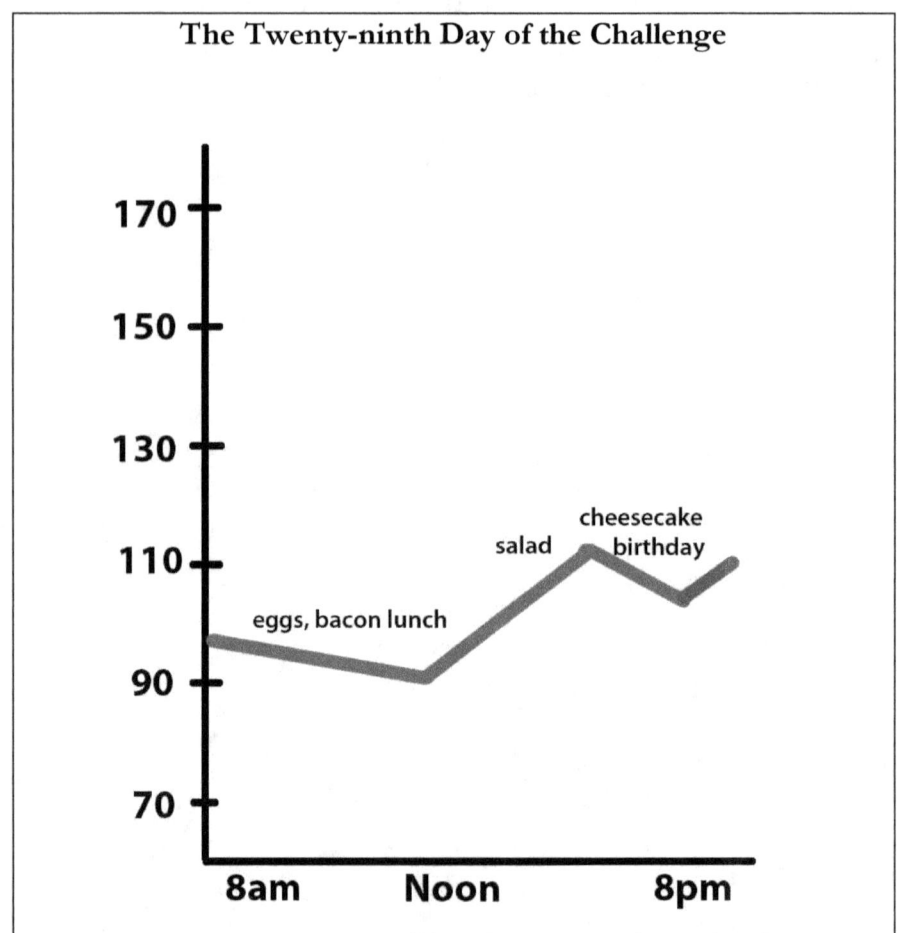

The Twenty-ninth Day of the Challenge

(graph showing blood sugar levels throughout the day)

170
150
130
110 — salad — cheesecake birthday
eggs, bacon lunch
90
70

8am   Noon   8pm

Officially I have lost 8 pounds since August 12. I ate breakfast late while visiting a relative in Zion at lunch. I tried cheesecake for our grandsons birthday. I started with a small piece and added another. An hour later my sugar was only 109! For the third time the omission of breakfast led to lower sugar all day. Is it a coincidence or a trend?

.

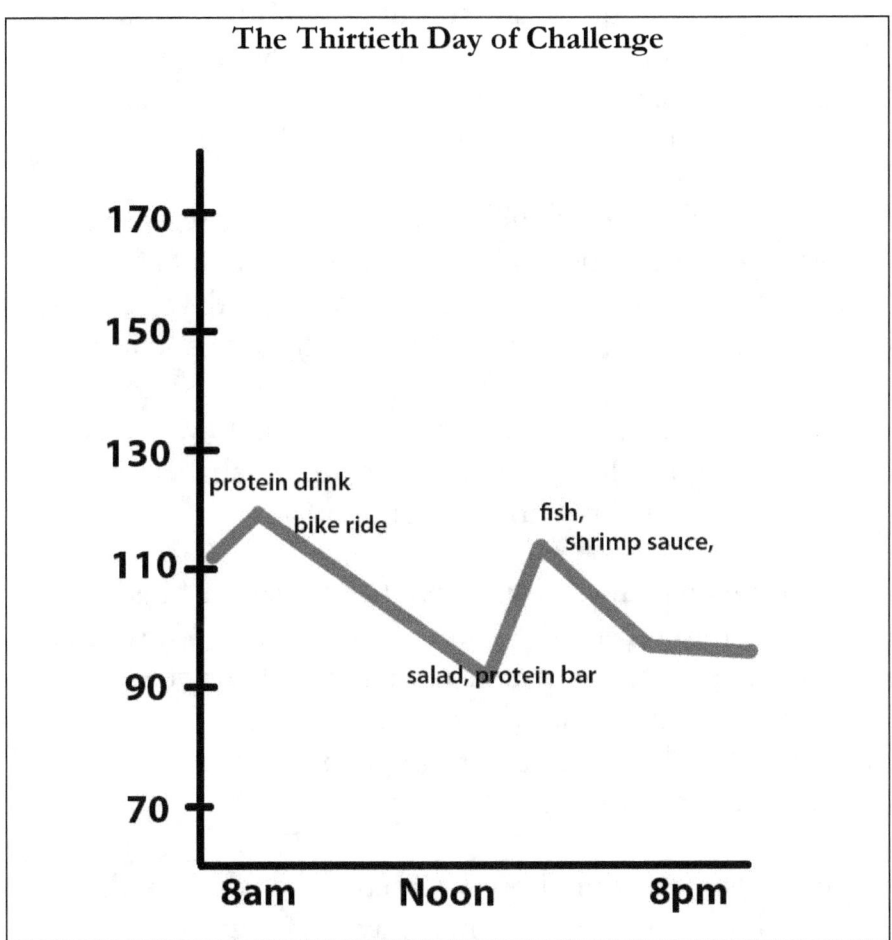

The Thirtieth Day of Challenge

170
150
130
protein drink
bike ride
fish,
shrimp sauce,
110
salad, protein bar
90
70

8am   Noon   8pm

This is the last day of my 30 day challenge. The glucose readings today are consistent with what I would expect based on exercise and food selection. My blood sugar did not rise in spite of having a protein drink at breakfast time. There were no excessive spikes or troughs and still no insulin. Perhaps my muscles are more sensitive to insulin and using glucose efficiently.

I maintained frequent daily testing for another 30 days. My diet consisted of the foods that maintained steady sugars in the past. I did not have to add insulin again. My charts remained relatively flat, between 90 and 120.

Looking back, it seems like I resolved the diabetes in a short time. While the challenge was in process it seemed like a very long time. After these first thirty days my blood sugar readings became very predictable and static. Blood sugars two hours after meals are usually below 140 and 75% of morning readings are 110 or below. I never began taking insulin again after this 30 day challenge. I recently discarded my unused supply.

The entire challenge would have been easier if I had made the connection to total carbohydrates earlier. I was under the impression from diabetic authorities that sweet potatoes, whole grains and most vegetables were acceptable. I believe they prolonged my loosely controlled diabetes for eight years.

I began using sprouted bread based on my daughter's successful diet program. It may have made some difference in sugar response based on my challenge

Chapter Four

The Numbers

...A simple graph in my lab report would have clearly indicated an upward trajectory in the years prior to my diagnosis...

1999-2008, Prior to my Type 2 Diabetic Diagnosis

Fortunately, I have maintained hard copies of my lab results for years. After review, I found in 1999 my fasting glucose on a routine lab report was 78. In 2002, my fasting glucose was 89. In 2005 it was 99. In 2006, it was 103. It was on a move upward but not yet diabetes. In November of 2007 it was 106, past borderline, and should have alerted my physician. He noted on the report, concern with liver enzymes and cholesterol at the time, but no mention of the glucose. In March of 2008 my fasting sugar reached 122. The physician commented again on abnormal cholesterol needing treatment, but not about the glucose.

Only eight months later, in November 2008, when I saw a new doctor and was clearly diabetic, my fasting sugar was 303. It had doubled in the preceding six months.

I remember looking in the mirror and observing a gray appearance in my face during this time. I wondered if I was sick but I had no symptoms of high blood glucose. I did drink a lot of water and my waist line had expanded during this time.

A simple graph in my lab report would have clearly indicated an upward trajectory in the years prior to my diagnosis. My experience also reveals how quickly type 2 diabetes can accelerate.

My fasting glucose had more than doubled in six months but I did not feel symptoms of high blood sugar. I had become used to it.

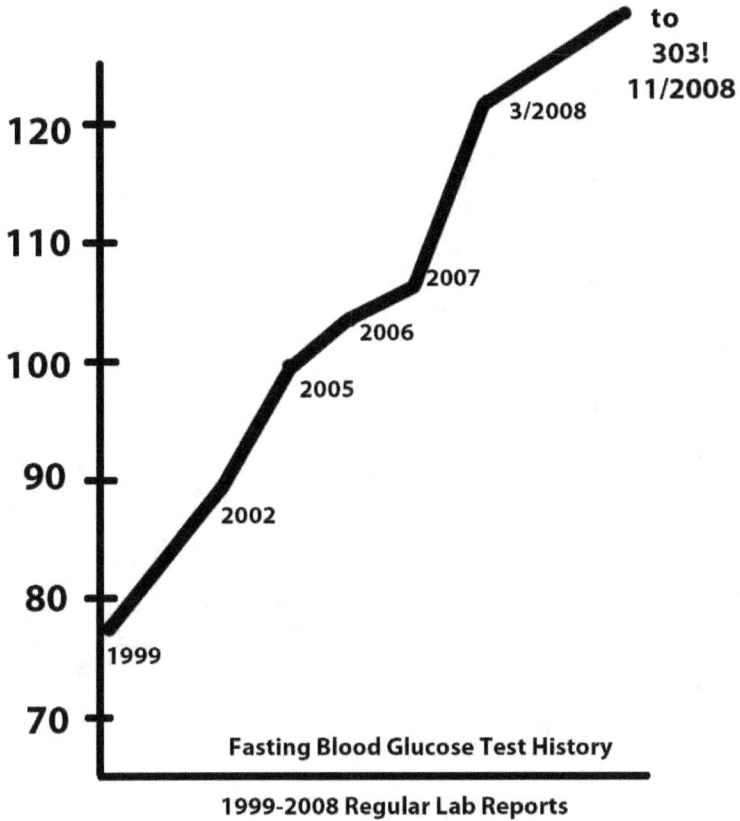

Fasting Blood Glucose Test History

1999-2008 Regular Lab Reports

After Initial Diagnosis- November 2008

I found my original blood sugar personal record book for the first days after being diagnosed with diabetes. The daily self testing blood sugar results are frightening. I had begun a rigid diet based on the information that I had and I was using oral anti-glycemic medicine for the first ten days before I switched to insulin.

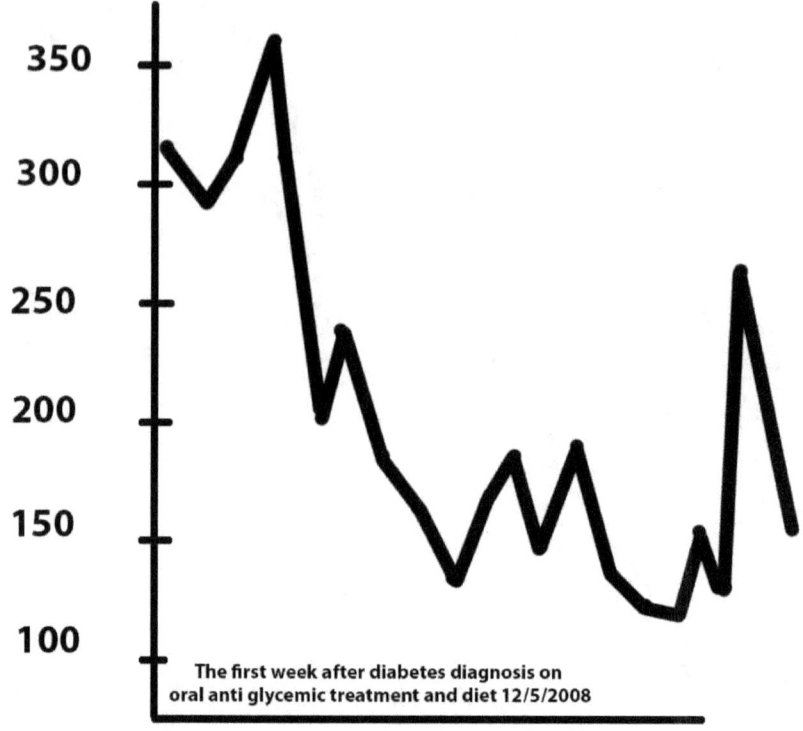

The first week after diabetes diagnosis on oral anti glycemic treatment and diet 12/5/2008

As with every challenge in my diabetes history, the remedy seems to need three days to take effect. From the third day to the tenth day there was a remarkable reduction. Since that time, the levels remained relatively constant for years until I began my Charting Challenge.

My early blood sugar readings after insulin initiation in 2008 reveal a baseline that is too high and dramatic spikes. Too frequent meals, eating before blood sugar had dropped normally and large portions probably explain the spikes. There was no improvement in my condition, and it actually worsened in future years according to my A1C chart.

The A1C blood test measures the average blood sugar over the prior three months. In non-diabetics the A1C is usually below 5.5, in diabetics commonly over 6.0.

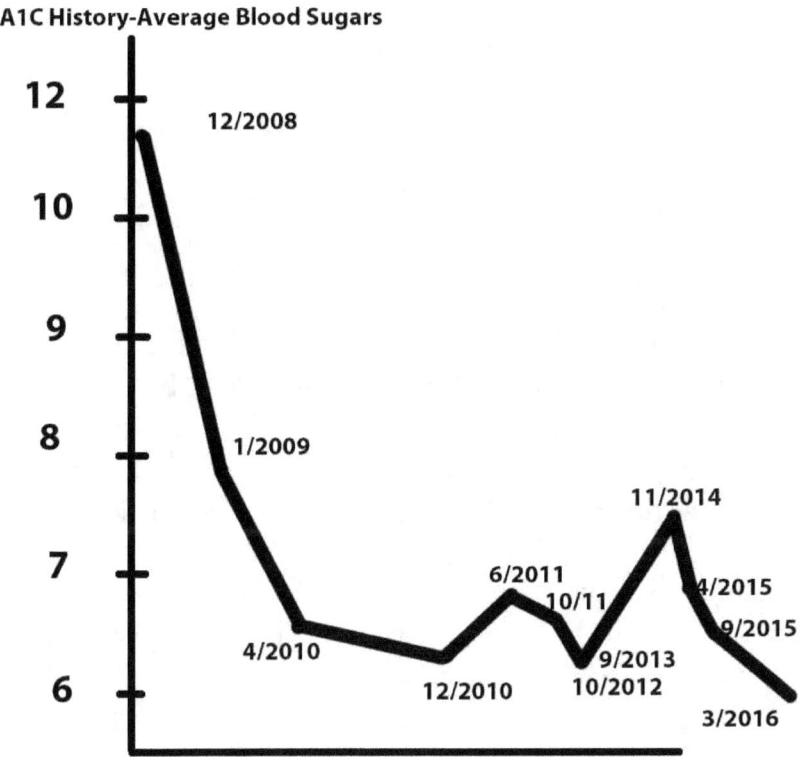

A1C History-Average Blood Sugars

Interpreting A1C scores
5% = average sugar 97
6% = average sugar 126
7% = average sugar 154
8% = average sugar 183
9% = average sugar 212
10% = average sugar 240
11% = average sugar 269
12% = average sugar 298

The situation did not change until I was motivated by the promise and had to find my own solution. I knew that prior trials and recommendations were insufficient. The charting allowed me objective measures for food selection and meal timing. It allowed me to take control.

Diabetic authorities had called foods with less than 5 grams of carbohydrates, "free" foods. *What is that saying, There is no such thing as a free lunch?*

As I stated I tried to limit carbohydrates to 50 grams a day. A diabetic authority suggests 60 grams a meal for women with 5 servings of fruit or vegetables, 3 whole grains and three low fat dairy selections. *Perhaps this works for some people, I would be enormous if I ate like this.*

Chapter Five

Since My Charting Challenge

Six months later...

As of March 2016 I have maintained a 16 pound loss of weight. I believe the smaller portions was a result of the higher protein meals that are very filling. I didn't realize until January that my challenge diet was in effect a low carb diet.

The easiest diet for me to follow to keep my sugar low and my weight off was a breakfast menu, excluding the toast, potatoes or pancakes. Eggs, with cheese, sausage and bacon had little effect on my blood sugar. In recent weeks, I have been able to occasionally eat a sandwich or popcorn without significant sugar effects. I still cannot tolerate rice, beans, yogurt or oat meal.

I have not consistently tested my sugar throughout the day since the first 60 days. However, I have been consistently monitoring my fasting sugar levels which have remained below 110 in 75% of my tests.

Recent Sampling of Fasting Blood Glucose

March to May 2016

113	105
104	119
124	119
98	100
104	109
113	90
110	122
110	78
108	108
104	118
102	88
97	95
101	110
90	110
102	85
120	105

92	105
78	122

If I had to repeat the challenge I would have gradually reduced the insulin to avoid stopping and restarting and the sudden spikes or troughs in my sugar. If I had to repeat the challenge, I would have informed my physician also.

I have begun adding mineral supplements to my daily vitamins. The changes in my diet have affected my potassium level slightly, which is low but still within normal limits. This may be due to the avoidance of all potatoes which are a strong source of potassium.

Eight months later...

I tried adding rice to my meals. At the first attempt I fell asleep for three hours and then measured my glucose, it was 170. Still defiant, I also tried oatmeal, my glucose rose for three hours, finally reaching 160.

The Next Six Months

I intend to renew my efforts through smaller portions and carbohydrate restriction to lose another sixteen pounds. I expect that my A1C will drop to 5.5 or below on my next test. The problem of family celebrations and social events is still an issue. I choose not to participate in most events where I cannot control the food choices. Eventually I hope I can control my appetite. I am finding it easier to engage in conversation without eating or drinking.

I have not experienced any symptoms from limiting my carbs, although I sometimes consume more than 50 grams a day.

If I became non diabetic what would my blood sugar be? I did some research and found the answer is up in the air. Generally non diabetics have sugar levels 70-108 after fasting overnight. After meals non diabetics have sugar 70-140.

A1C Reductions Long Term Sugar Control

April to September 2015- a .4 reduction in A1C 6.8 to 6.4

My A1C was reduced from 6.8 in March 2015 to 6.4 in September 2015. I was disappointed at the time based on the significant changes I had made in my diet. The diet changes were begun July 28 2015.

September 2015 to March 2016 - another .4 reduction in A1C 6.4 to 6.0

The period between September and March was relatively easy. I started to regain a couple pounds and my fasting sugar level increased between November and January. In January 2016, after reading a carbohydrate diet book, I realized that my diet selection based on my blood sugar test was effectively a low carb diet. Choosing foods then became easier when I could follow the low carb labels in the stores. I had previously read that carrots, romaine lettuce, beets, peas, beans were "free" foods. However, three leaves of romaine lettuce have 1 gram of carbohydrate.

Results Still Rely on Accountability

I calculated my fasting sugar levels after ten days over four periods.

- In late November my average fasting sugar was 108.1.
- In early February it had risen to 121.7.
- In late February my ten day fasting sugar was only 98.7 when I resumed closer monitoring.
- In mid March it had risen slightly to 101.7

I realized that I had failed to maintain strict adherence or testing because I had not seen my doctor since September. Accountability is very important. I scheduled another doctor's appointment and it motivated me to renew my efforts to control my diet and sugar.

Weight, Portions and Low Carbohydrate is My Answer

Was the lower sugar the result of smaller portions, total weight loss, or change of diet? I can only guess based on my personal experience. I found the total carbohydrate diet is my personal solution. The bread, rice, yogurt, fruits, and the potatoes affect on my sugar are explained by the level of total carbohydrates. This challenge would have been simpler if I had known this when I began.

The carbohydrate connection was not apparent previously because I had been told that some high carb foods were acceptable, like sweet potatoes and whole grains.

When I shop for groceries it is based on the total carbohydrate content. Most soups and packaged convenience foods are too high in carbohydrates for my diet.

I recently read diet advice, don't eat when you are not hungry. It seems so simple and yet life gets it the way.

I try to maintain about 50 grams of carbohydrate a day. Some days I succeed.

Eggs, cheese, fish and meat and oils have little or no carbohydrate and little effect on my sugar levels. The only dairy product I use is cream in my coffee. Cream has 10 grams in 8 ounces. Eggs have half a gram of carbohydrate, beef, pork, chicken, turkey and fish have no carbohydrate. Cheeses vary from .2 to 1 gram per Tablespoon. Peanut butter has 8 grams in 2 Tablespoons. I buy low carb varieties of bread that contain 14 grams or less per slice. I keep frozen brussel sprouts at 11 grams, broccoli and peas. I also sometimes have a glass of wine with less than 4 gram of carbs.

The following are carbohydrate contents of ordinary foods. The carb content should be checked on the product package. I have found wide ranges in carbs.

Pretzels (10)   47

Dry Roasted Peanuts (39) 5

Black beans ½ cup	32
Oatmeal ½ cup	27
Rye crackers (5)	44
Butter crackers (5)	51
White Flour (1 cup)	95
Whole grain flour	86
Quinoa 1/4 cup	29
Rice 1 cup	50
Brown Rice (1/2 cup)	35
Sweet potato	22
White potato, small	15
Pasta 1/2 cup	19
Brown Rice Spaghetti	43
Egg noodles 1/2 cup	18
Cashews 1/4 cup	9
Apple	21
Banana	23
Pear	25

Beer (12 ounce)   13

Popcorn (3 TB

        unpopped)   25

Half and Half 2 TB   1

As I previously mentioned, some diabetic authorities recommended fruits, beans, oatmeal and whole grain breads for patients. My charting revealed the negative consequences on my sugar before I realized that carbohydrates were a valid indicator.

I have not found net carbs to have less effect on my blood sugar. I have not found low glycemic index foods to have less effect on my blood sugar either. Perhaps this is because I overindulged, thinking they were "free" foods?

The reader may be interested in the carbohydrate content of obvious poor choices. Knowing the carb counts can be sufficient to avoid the craving;

Angel food cake slice   29

Chocolate cake   38

Dark chocolate (1 oz)   18

Doughnut   26

Cherry pie   69

Apple pie   57

| Pecan pie | 67 |
| Pumpkin pie | 40 |

I have stopped drinking even one beer because of the carbohydrate content. Instead, I sometimes have a glass of red wine with dinner which I found does limit the glucose response to a meal.

Exercise and Weights

I can observe the effect of workout with weights on my charts. When I feel the familiar back of my neck aching from high sugar weight lifting will usually resolve it. The effect of biking is not as consistent. I have continued to use weights to counter high sugars and excess eating. I have increased the weight load by 50% in recent weeks. Weight lifting on a daily basis has probably compensated for the omission of daily insulin. I am lifting 70 pounds on most machines. I avoid the overhead weight lift to avoid shoulder injury.

Eating Out Again When Necessary

There are nutrition labels available on the internet for popular restaurant options. I have memorized a few and they are applicable to many restaurants. A slice of thin crust pizza is roughly 30 grams of carbs. Chicken nuggets are, as I suspected, the best option. A six piece is about 15 grams of carbohydrate with no sauce.

It is the sandwich buns that raise the carbohydrate content. Cheeseburgers, lunchmeat sandwiches on hoagie rolls and chicken sandwiches contain 30-45 grams of carbohydrates. Soft serve milk shakes are as bad as I thought, about 75- 100 grams.

A baked potato with sour cream as a side is about 60 grams, 50% more than fries.

Protein and fat eaten at the same time with carbohydrates is supposed to limit the impact of the carbohydrate. I tested the theory with popcorn and butter and didn't find a significant difference.

I was correct in my self testing that Mexican and Asian meals were high in carbohydrates. Nachos are about 30 grams of carbohydrates, burritos about 60, and a single taco, 15. A cup of rice is about 50 grams and many Asian main dishes are also sweetened.

An Ordinary Type 2 Diabetic Patient's Advice to Diabetes Educators

Diabetes educators need to update their diet recommendations for type 2 diabetics. They should recognize the carbohydrate impact and be less concerned about overall health. For type 2 diabetics it is all about the sugar levels. We can supplement with vitamins and minerals and monitor for reduction in fruits, legumes and many vegetables.

These are some of the other practical diabetic issues for newly diagnosed type 2 patients that I never found addressed during the past eight years;

- What is an acceptable range of blood sugar spikes up and down? What is considered dangerous?

- Is the range more important than the average?
- What blood sugar numbers do other diabetic patients experience?
- What is the potential blood sugar effect of foods and how soon does it happen?
- When does the effect of a bad food choice diminish?
- How much does exercise effect sugars? What about strenuous exercise?
- What happens if I skip a meal? Sometimes I don't feel like eating.
- How effective is the different types of insulin either long or short acting? How do I decide which to use?
- Is diet more important or effective than insulin?
- How much and what type of insulin is used typically?
- How frequently can I adjust the insulin dose or stop using it entirely?

The best diabetes education resource I found was <u>Dr. Bernstein's Diabetes Solution: A Complete Guide to Achieving Normal Blood Sugars</u>[2].   It is especially useful because Dr. Bernstein is a type 1 diabetic and shares his personal experience. He challenges diabetes educators and authorities to toughen the blood sugar goals for diabetics.

---

[2] .Richard K Bernstein, MD, <u>Dr Bernstein's Diabetes Solution: A Complete Guide to Achieving Normal Blood Sugars</u>, Little, Brown and Co., 1997

The Hard Truth for Bad Patients Like Me

I have type 2, not type 1 diabetes and I recognize that my dietary habits created the condition. Like most type 2 diabetics, I have somewhat out of control sugars and am somewhat overweight.

I admit I am a pathetic and stubborn patient with a curable lifestyle driven disease. I put myself in this condition and it is my effort that can bring me back to normal blood sugars. No medicine, individual physician, diabetes diet, or educational program can do it.

It is our personal D-day battle against our personal weakness.

An Example to Improve Upon

Copy the following page to start your own diary:

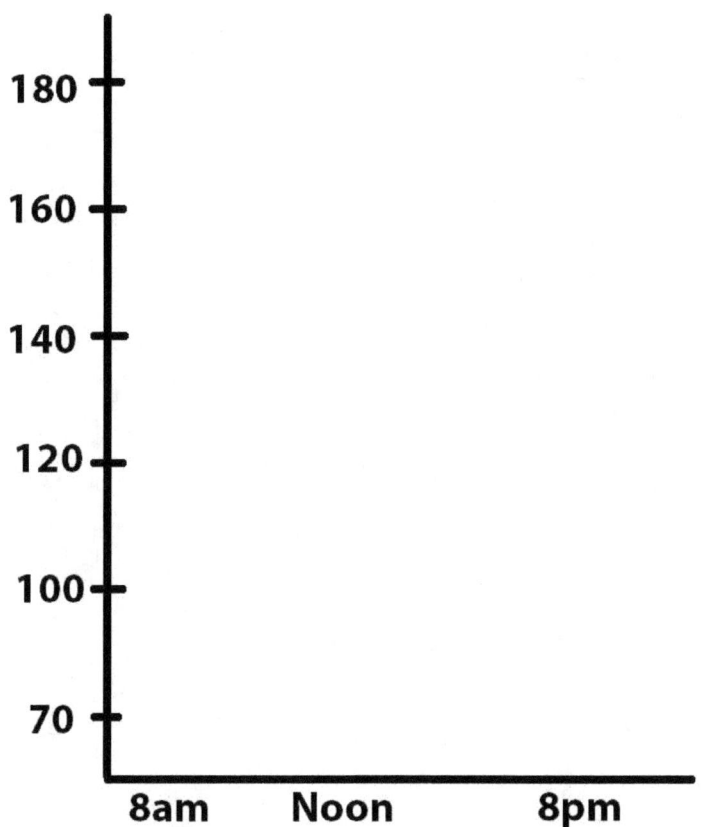

Date:

Notes:

Exercise:

Diet:

Stress:

www.ingramcontent.com/pod-product-compliance
Lightning Source LLC
Chambersburg PA
CBHW071217280526
45787CB00002B/711